Ending The Sex Wars

Ending The Sex Wars

✦

A Woman's Guide to Understanding Men

Dr. Morley D. Glicken

Professor Emeritus, California State University,

San Bernardino

And

Executive Director, The Institute for Positive Growth:

A Training, Research, and Consulting Cooperative

Los Angeles, California

iUniverse, Inc.

New York Lincoln Shanghai

Ending The Sex Wars
A Woman's Guide to Understanding Men

iUniverse books may be ordered through booksellers or by contacting:

iUniverse
2021 Pine Lake Road, Suite 100
Lincoln, NE 68512
www.iuniverse.com
1-800-Authors (1-800-288-4677)

ISBN-13: 978-0-595-36007-9 (pbk)
ISBN-13: 978-0-595-80458-0 (ebk)
ISBN-10: 0-595-36007-6 (pbk)
ISBN-10: 0-595-80458-6 (ebk)

Printed in the United States of America

Contents

Preface

This book about men is written to help women understand the often strange and perplexing behavior of the men in their lives. There's no reason men might not read it as well since the book is written to help men and women get along better. If it's true that we have a sex war going on, then all of us lose by not making peace and getting on with the pleasant task of loving and enjoying each other.

This book is a practical guide, but for readers who want something more academic, a book I wrote entitled <u>Working with Troubled Men: A Contemporary Practitioner's Guide</u> (2005), written specifically for psychotherapists is available through Lawrence Erlbaum Publishers (http://www.erlbaum.com).

Parts of this book were written while I was living in Southern California and teaching at a university. I am now writing books full-time and serve as director of the Institute for Personal Growth: A Consulting, Research, and Training Cooperative serving people's needs that are often ignored by psychotherapists and the media. Men are one of those ignored areas of concern. I'm not sure why since men seem to be having their share of problems these days from lagging behind women in educational achievement, to having more health problems, and to significant amounts of alcoholism drug abuse, crime, and violence. When men do badly, we all suffer. So, for the reader who makes this journey into the world of men, God bless and good journey.

Dr. Morley D. Glicken

1

Men: The Endangered Species

Coffee Shop Wisdom

Most mornings I go to a local cafe in Southern California for coffee. It's a sort of ritual for me. Sometimes I write checks for bills I owe or read the dismal news in the paper while other times I try and organize my day or grade the accumulated papers I must read as a professor of social work at a California university.

The local men often walk by my table and nod in recognition. Sometimes they stop and talk to me about my articles in the local papers about men. These men are the workingmen of America; the plumbers and construction workers, the common laborers and retired railroad workers, the illegal immigrants from Mexico. Their trucks and beat up old cars line the parking lot outside of the restaurant.

I have come to value my conversations with these men. Many of them have done badly by women and children, and readily admit it. Some of them are extraordinary people who have done better than most of us. And there are always the men who sit and talk about women and you want to get up and ream them out. They sound like abusers. Worse, they sound like children in adult bodies.

I've learned a lot from listening and talking to these men in the morning. Academics and therapists hear pretty unrealistic versions of life, but these men talk like real people. People with flaws. Human beings we all know in our daily lives.

When the wives and children of these men talk to me, you get a different picture of their behavior. They talk about abuse and neglect, about put downs and absences, and sometimes, about abandonment. They describe, in detail, how the insensitive behavior of their men affects the women and children who are trying so hard to love their husbands, boy friends, and fathers.

Sometimes I get a chance to sit with the men and women and listen to them talk about the gender wars they have fought. The men often sit with their mouths open and ask, "Was I that bad?" Everybody nods their heads. The men have mellowed so it isn't easy for them to imagine that they've acted so badly in the past.

Sometimes the men hang around, after the women leave, to assure me that they weren't so bad, but there's an emptiness to their denial that rings hollow. Many times they walk away shaking their head, angry at me for making them hear so much bad stuff about behavior they'd rather forget, mean, nasty, hurtful behavior which has been like a knife in the hearts of the women and children trying so hard to understand them.

The men who interrupt me as I try and drink my coffee are ordinary men. Men who have had troubles in their lives, men who drink too much, from time to time, and men who can be mean and petty. They're the men who regret their past and have done a thing or two that leave them in the night sweats when they awake from bad dreams. Normal men who have made mistakes. Decent guys who cared for the baby at night and provide for families when it was nearly impossible.

Sensitive men? Probably not. Romantic men? I doubt it. Men who sweep women off their feet with the power and brilliance of their lovemaking? It doesn't seem very likely. Just regular "Joes" who need the guidance and the sweet and tender loving of a woman. Men who are better when a woman is in their life. Men who can hardly navigate the complexities of life and who depend on women in ways that are sometimes childlike.

Men like Roger, a plumber, who joins the early morning construction gang at my coffee shop. He sees me sitting in the back reading the paper and comes over to sit with me. Today he complains about his wife. She's too fat, he says. He's lost interest in her. I look over at Roger, who is perhaps 60 or 70 pounds overweight, and I ask if he's looked in the mirror lately. Does he know that his obesity is as off-putting to his wife as hers is to him? He mumbles something derogatory about my mother, but I see him everyday and he looks somehow, thinner. When I see him weeks later with his wife, they look nice together. Warm, maybe even tender in the way older men and women can be with each another.

He doesn't thank me for my advice or say how much his life has improved because of my simple suggestions. All he does is bring his wife over, an attractive woman in her forties, while I drink my coffee and try and read the paper. He beams at me. See how great my wife looks, his smile says? See what a hunk I must be to attract such a great looking lady? It is thanks enough and I smile at their happiness.

Another guy, Richard, one of the few Black men who sit in the cafe, complains to me about the way his wife spends his money. "She's a shopping junky," he says. "Ain't no way anyone can spend so much money."

He brings her in one morning, a nice, soft-spoken young woman. She talks to me about how difficult it is for a Black family to make ends meet, but Richard is a good husband and father and they make the money go a little further. Richard wants to buy me breakfast. He feels like dancing in the cafe. His wife has touched a part of his heart with love seeds.

How strange men must seem to women. How they talk so badly about the women in their lives but depend on them for everything. And how badly men do in giving women credit for so much that women do to make their lives easier. And yet women are there to help in the small and large ways that men almost never regard as important or admit make a difference.

How absolutely contradictory male behavior must seem to most women. How men prance, and strut, and brag without end when inside they often feel as inadequate as anyone can feel and still get manage to get up in the morning and put their clothes on. And yet to talk to them, men seem on top of the world, kings of the hill, beyond pain.

Were it only so. If men were so secure, they wouldn't do the often-terrible things they do to wives, girlfriends, co-workers and children. They wouldn't abuse and abandon their loved ones, or fly into jealous rages, or harass women in the workplace. If men were the winners in this war among the genders, they wouldn't fall apart in mid-life, or suffer the indignity of bodies, which fail them and leave them old and emotionally wrecked well before God meant for such a thing to happen.

Just as I talk to the men when I have coffee in the mornings, I have come to cherish the time I spend talking to the women I see who come in for a quick cup of coffee before their impossibly long and complicated days begin. They are the workingwomen of America, the unglamorous women who get up at 5 AM and care for their families before driving an hour or more to thankless jobs. I have come to think of these women as very special people. They have been the prisoners in the war among the sexes. Though they are often battered and war weary, they still have an optimism about the flawed men they often meet, fall in love with, and marry.

They are the women like Betty Sue who, early one morning asks me what to do when a man loses interest in sex. As I begin to talk to her, some of the women in the coffee shop join us.

"He's a good man," she says, "and we used to have a great love life. I'm sure something is really wrong."

One of the women in the group sitting at the table says, "Why not just say to him something like, 'Honey, it sure used to be nice how we'd spend our time in bed. It would sure be nice to have that again.' Why not give it a try?" Betty Sue looks over at me and I nod in support.

The next day she comes back with a big smile on her face. All of the ladies at the table rib her until she says, "He thought I wasn't interested anymore. He thought maybe I was with another man, and it was making him crazy."

"How could he think something like that?" someone asks, and one of the ladies says, "Because, he's a man. That's the way men think."

Another time, Denise, a woman perhaps in her late thirties is going through the early stages of knowing that her marriage is all but over. "I don't understand it, doc," she says to me. "We were such good friends. We really liked being together. But now, he just always seems like he's in another world. When we talk, it's always about the house or the car, it's never about how unhappy we are together."

It's very early in the morning but Denise has been up for hours and her blood-shot eyes suggest that she's been crying in the car on the way to the coffee shop. "It's tough," I tell her, "when a man shuts off. Have you asked him if something is wrong at work or in his personal life?"

She shakes her head. "He always tells me when something is wrong," she says. "He's not one to keep things inside."

We sit in silence for a while and watch the regulars walk in, many of them still sleepy from nights too short to make up for the hours of driving and the hard work ahead of them. I look at Denise and gently touch her hand. "Maybe there's something wrong, Denise, that's so troubling to your husband that he can't discuss it with you. Men often find it hard to talk about really personal problems. Try asking him tonight and stay with it. Don't let him slough you off or avoid talking."

Denise looks at me with a look I've seen all too often. The moment comes in a relationship when you've tried everything and you've unconsciously begun to give up. It's the moment of being psychologically divorced. Denise looks up and nods her head, her shoulders slumped. "O.K. doc," she says, "I'll try for you, but I don't think it's gonna work."

A week goes by and Denise hasn't come in for coffee. I'm all too ready to blame myself for bad advice since failure is an occupational hazard we live with in the helping professions. But one morning she comes in with her husband. They find their way over to my booth and after introductions and handshakes, Denise and her husband, Ed, sit for a while and drink their coffee while we make small talk. Finally, Denise tells me what's happened in the past week with Ed looking on, a serious look on his face.

"I didn't want to do it, doc, but I knew you'd be hurt if I came to you for advice and didn't use it. So I waited until Ed was sitting in his chair after dinner and I made the kids go outside so we could talk. I said to Ed how he seems to be unhappy all the time and that I don't think we're gonna make it. And he says back to me that he's fine and that it's my imagination. But I won't let it go, doc, and I kept at it until he finally says to me that he thinks he might lose his job and he doesn't think I'll stay with him if he doesn't have a job."

I look over at Ed and he's nodding quietly as Denise tells the story. We pause for a moment to drink our coffee and then Denise continues.

"Where did he get that crazy idea? I asked him and he says, 'from you, Denise, from you.' I argued with him about that but he reminded me of the many times I've said, sarcastically, that I'd never take care of a man. And it's true. I've said it a lot but I didn't mean <u>my</u> man. But of course, that's the way he took it. We talked most of the week about the situation and we got it straightened up. We didn't think we could because there were so many other things that were going wrong, but we did and it's so much better now I can't even believe it was possible. I thought that Ed was like most men and that he couldn't talk about the really tough stuff. He fooled me, though. Once I reached out a little, he could talk just fine."

I've had hundreds of conversations like this with the men and women of the coffee shop. Not all of them end so dramatically or well, but I think that men and women are much better together with a little gentle guidance, some good information, and some timely help.

One morning the women at the coffee shop ask if I've ever thought about writing a simple book about men written for women. Many of them have benefited from our discussions over coffee and feel that other women might also benefit. What they ask for is a book with the stories about women and men that I've accumulated in over 30 years as a teacher and therapist. They also ask for simple explanations about the way men behave and how women might deal more successfully with men.

After the suggestion kicked around inside my head for sometime, I asked my 18-year-old daughter, Amy, what she thought about the idea. "What do you know about women, dad?" she said. Humility is always a good way to approach any project, so I told her, "Not much, but I think I know a lot about men. How about I write what I know about men and you help me put it in a way that won't make women want to come after me with pitch forks."

Actually, I said this same thing to a number of friends and colleagues and to the men and women I see regularly at the coffee shop. They all kindly consented.

My promise to you, the reader, is to include the stories I've heard about men and women in over 30 years as a therapist and professor of social work. I've included a story or two about my family and the often mysterious and wonderful happenings in my home life while growing up in a small town in North Dakota. I'll try not to talk psychobabble or to give you advice that makes you feel instinctively that I'm talking nonsense.

If the book works for you, then men won't be such a mystery, although it's true that men aren't always easy to understand. Our behavior is often based upon codes of conduct and beliefs that even we men don't fully understand. I'll try to explain those codes of conduct and beliefs so that you can enjoy the men in your life.

I think men and women hunger for better times. No one wants to be in a constant war between the sexes. When relationships between men and women improve, we all gain. And since love is everything it's cracked up to be nothing in this world beats the wonder of two people in love.

In developing the book, I've asked many people about the content. Most wanted me to concentrate on the way men handle relationships and the problems men have in marriage. I've done just that by including chapters on love, marriage, divorce, single life and on the dangerous men women sometimes meet who can be terribly abusive. I've also included material on men's health, men and crisis, old age and the problems of men of color. And no book on men would be complete without a word or two about the workplace, that battle zone where men can act like warriors, where no prisoners are taken and where men channel their warrior philosophies into winning, at any cost.

So here goes. Let's discover what we can about men to make your life just a little easier and maybe in the process, their life, as well.

2

The Five Minute Primer on Why Men Act So Strangely

Judy, one of the regulars at the coffee shop, comes up to me one morning and asks if she can talk to me. Judy is a working woman up early in the morning and, like so many women in this area of southern California where I live, about to drive two hours to her job in Los Angeles. Maybe it's 6:00 AM and Judy will have to hit the road in a few minutes to get to work by 8:30. The roads this time of day are clogged. Judy will fight the same traffic problems on the way home.

"Hey, it's a job," she tells me as we drink our coffee together. "I feel lucky to have a job. Most women in my position are on welfare. No thanks," she says, but she has two boys who rarely see their father and the boys are starting to get into trouble at school. She tries to keep them in line by being strict, but being latchkey children, like so many children in America, she doesn't have much control over their lives while she's at work and, of course, her ex-husband doesn't help.

"They're starting to act like the old man," she says. "The same bad attitude. I don't seem to be able to make them understand that they're going to get into trouble, just like their dad got into trouble when he was in school. They think that's what boys are supposed to do."

I listen and nod my head in recognition. I've often heard this story from the single mothers out there trying their best to raise kids alone.

"I don't understand men," Judy says with a sound of resignation in her voice. "They seem to belong to some club where they all decide to act the same way even if it gets them into trouble all of their lives. Stubborn, that's what they are. Plain stubborn like mules. You try to tell them things about life and they look at you like you're crazy. They think they know better, of course, because they're men."

In the next few minutes before she hits the road, I give Judy a crash course on understanding why men act the way they do, even her young sons.

The Crazy, Troubled, Nutty, Violent World of Men

No one knows for sure why men behave the way they do, I tell Judy. Maybe it has to do with hormonal differences. Possibly, from the past, men are genetically prepared to be warriors and hunters, which might explain our aggressive nature. Perhaps the way men are taught to be men, the process of socialization explains why men tend to be very different from women. We are, after all, taught to be tough-minded and action-oriented no matter what the cost is to others.

And we know that men tend to be less sensitive to the feelings of others. Men are much more likely to handle situations with anger and confrontation than compromise and conciliation. Men hardly ever seek advice or help from others. That includes not asking directions when driving to not getting needed help for medical and emotional problems.

While no one sits down with young boys and teaches them a male code of conduct, most boys probably know the code by the time they're six, or earlier, and they live by it. They know, for example, that men who give into pain are sissies and that after a certain age, you never cry, ever. Men know that to not compete is a sign of weakness. Whatever the situation might be, there is an expectation that men will try and outdo one another. Not be competitive or to win at almost any cost is a sure sign that you're not a real man. No man wants other men to think that they are unmanly.

Adult men know that poor performance in sex is something to keep hidden from others. When men discuss sex, it's always to brag about their capacities and their conquests. Men know that sensitivity to others and the ability to look at the motives for their behavior (let's call that introspection), are feminine qualities. If you show those qualities to other men, you might get ridiculed.

Many of the messages men first learn are given in sports. Here, men are taught about winning and superiority. Brannon (1976) believes that there are four primary messages given to all men at an early age and that sports and the play of young boys help young men master these messages. They are:

1. No sissy stuff: the need to be different from women.
2. The big weed: the need to be superior to others.
3. The sturdy oak: the need to be self-reliant and independent.
4. Give em Hell: the need to be more powerful than others, through violence, if necessary.

Boys who have unstable home lives or who have problems learning these messages in socially acceptable ways learn exaggerated male behavior. Tiller (1967) calls this process, "compensatory masculinity." It describes boys striving to become men who feel fearful and insecure about themselves while they learn to be men. To deal with their insecurities, these boys may drink, smoke, use drugs, or exercise their power over others at an early age to exaggerate their need to be seen as real men. Men who are abusive in their relationships with women and children often suffer from compensatory masculinity.

To make sure that Judy better understands the four main messages that boys learn as they become men, I suggest to Judy that I explain how these messages are taught starting with, "No sissy stuff."

1. No Sissy Stuff: The Need to be Different From Women. Boys are taught to be different from girls almost immediately. Parents, who try and encourage boys to be sensitive and to recognize their feminine side often fight an uphill battle. Older boys teach younger boys to be tough, invulnerable, and independent. Movies and television reinforce that lesson.

Older men subtly influence boys to be unemotional when they hurt. No pain, no gain. Boys play hurt in sports and make pain a symbol of their manliness. Where boys are taught to control and deny their feelings, girls are taught to express them. Watch a sporting match sometime, I tell Judy, and see how many of the male players are not only playing hurt but are actually getting rewarded by their teammates for their behavior.

"But that's crazy stuff," Judy complains. "They should stop and see a doctor."

"Sure they should," I respond, "but if they do that the other boys and the older men will think they're sissies. So they play hurt even if it ruins their career or results in a serious injury or health problem. "Furthermore," I tell her, "as boys mature into young men, this message becomes a code of conduct. 'If you can't stand the heat, get out of the kitchen.' Think of the messages we pass on to young men. They are messages of strength and endurance, of mastery of pain, of bravery and selflessness. They are the warrior codes that men learn early in life.

Judy's son Tim, a ten year old confirms what I've said one Saturday morning as he joins Judy for breakfast. He's a nice boy, not at all the way Judy has described him. But then he's on his best behavior, I suppose. He says: "If you let them get away with anything then they think you're a girl. The names they call you are always girl's name. This boy I know at school, he backed down from a fight and everybody started calling him Edna and making kissing sounds. Pretty soon he got into a fight just to prove he was no baby, and he got beat up good. But all the guys were proud of him. And you know something? So were the girls, and he was proud of himself, too."

2. The Big Weed: The Need to be Superior to Others. Winning isn't something, said one of America's great coaches, it's everything. It isn't about wining or losing, said another coach, it's always about winning. And so it is. Boys know that being first, always winning, and being better than someone else is what men strive for. In sports, in work, in love. When women ask me why men have so few real male friends, it's hard to have friends, I tell them, when you're always competing with other men.

Judy tells me that her boys compete with one another all of the time. "It's like they're playing war games everyday. It drives me crazy. Who can eat the most, who knows more, who can get the bathroom first. They're always competing with each other. Even their father used to do the same with them when they were just little boys." I tell Judy about a former student who told a class I was teaching on men,

"I think women are as concerned about winning as men are. It's just that they have more subtle ways of showing it. Men are much more direct. You know that when men are together, somebody's going to get challenged. If you're out drinking, it'll be to see who can drink more or who can win at pool. It's always something. It's like the animals do when they carve out their territory by urinating around the boundaries. Men carve out their areas of superiority every time they interact with other men. But unlike women, it's direct confrontation, no guile allowed. Me against you, buddy. If you lose, then I'm the king of the hill."

Judy agrees. "Boy, it's enough to drive you nuts as a parent," she says.

Yes it is. It drives everybody nuts including the men who always have to prove themselves to others, including the women in their lives. Women, like men, learn the roles men are to play and enforce them as surely as men enforce expected male behavior on one another. All women? No, of course not. But most women learn gender roles early on in life and feel comfortable with the roles that apply to men.

3. The Sturdy Oak: The Need to be Self-reliant and Independent. By an early age, maybe three, when you observe young boys at play, you will notice that they often play alone. It tells you how well the culture trains its boys for independence.

Some developmental psychologists believe that men are biologically predisposed to be self-reliant and independent. Thousands of years of life as hunters and warriors have had an impact, they say, on the way men behave. Expecting men to be cooperative is not always part of the genetic imperative that drives male behavior. In the warrior cultures from which men come, these traits were necessary for survival. It's only been lately, perhaps in the past 50 years, that men have been criticized for being too self-reliant and too independent. Modern life demands cooperation, but men have been taught, in fact they are still taught, to be solitary players. Men resent supervision and control. "Give me a job," they tell you, "and let me do it." Listen to a conversation overheard at my favorite morning coffee spot among some construction workers.

"The foreman I had on the last job, he let us alone. Do your work, he says, be on time, get it done right. You know how to do it, so do it. We got the project done in no time. Got bonus points for getting it done early. It was great. We all felt like he respected us. But this guy we got now, he can't let anything happen without poking his big nose into it. One of the guys punched him out last week. They was gonna can him but the union saved him. Been a lot better on the job now, though, that's for sure. You gotta respect a man and leave him alone. Everybody knows that."

Judy shakes her head at this idea of independence and self-reliance. "Know it all's, that's what they are, know it all's. You can't tell men a damn thing," she says. "They know better and, even if they don't, they're gonna do it their way."

Probably. It takes a man a long time to learn that he can't do it all himself and that he often has to depend on others. By then, many men are in bad shape physically and emotionally from thinking that they have to do it all themselves. Healthy men learn to share and cooperate, troubled men don't.

4. <u>Give em Hell: The Need to be More Powerful Than Others Through Violence, if Necessary.</u> All boys are taught that if someone challenges you, you fight back. If you don't, it's a sign of weakness. To show weakness is not to be a man. Fights abound in the lives of young boys. This behavior continues on through adulthood. The stories men tell are all about giving the people around them, hell. I just heard this story from a colleague of mine in the university I work for, proving that education and rank don't stop men from giving people who cross them, hell.

"I was doing some consulting for a small school in the mid-west. I go out there every few months and the dean I was to work with torpedoed everything I did. I'd order something done and when I left, he'd counterman it. All he had was criticism for my work, but it was the kind that was petty and unimportant. Little put downs. Finally, we had a confrontation, really nasty. He actually threaten to fight me. I couldn't believe it. This little middle-aged guy, very academic, he actually wanted to duke it out with me. I stood up when he challenged me. I'm at least a foot taller and 50 pounds heavier but this guy stands up and makes a fist like he's going to hit me. Finally, I started to laugh and walked away. They removed him, of course, but it seemed so like our society. Even educated men, when everything else fails, resort to violence. It makes me wonder how far we've really come."

Judy looks as me for a long time. "Even educated men can act that way?" she asks.

"Who do you think start wars?" I ask her. "It's generally educated men with high social positions in the society. But they share, with all men, the common belief that if someone is pushing you around, that you have the right to push back, with a vengeance."

"But why do they act that way when it gets them into so much trouble?" she asks, glancing at her watch.

"Because," I respond, "it's about pride. Men would rather do something stupid like fighting than admit to themselves that someone got the best of them or that they were publicly humiliated. Men are very easy to read if you understand that pushing them around long enough will almost always result in the man pushing back."

"I gotta go, doc," she says. "I gotta hit the road and deal with all those macho men out there who drive like killers. But thanks, doc, it's been helpful," she says. "I got a lot to think about on the way to work."

She gets up and begins to walk toward the door but then she turns around and comes over and gives me a hug. It's a small gesture, but like all men who have pleased a woman a little bit, I am touched and go back to my work just a little happier than I was before.

What Does Male Socialization Mean For Women?

Men are often ruled by a code of conduct that may seem absurd and silly to women. It is absurd and silly, come to think of it, but it's very real to most men. That code of conduct has fierce repercussions in a man's world if it isn't followed. But the code of conduct can be modified and made more gentle in a good relationship. Women can soften men by using patience, kindness, and tact. A lot of all three, in fact.

Here's how to do it in love, work, and everyday life. Grab a cup of coffee and read each of these guidelines slowly and carefully. Then think about each one and try and see how you can apply each suggestion to your own life.

1) Respect the men in your life and demand the same of them. When men feel appreciated and respected, they're in a good place to return the favor. If they don't, then let them know what you want. Be direct, specific, and never expect more from them than you've asked. Men are, if nothing else, not very good at reading your minds. They're very concrete in the way they view the world. If you need more from them, tell them what you need.

2) Ask a man why he's doing something that troubles you. Very often when a man is able to discuss his behavior, he realizes that it doesn't make much sense and he may be open to suggestions. When a man asks for advice, give it to him. Be informative and give him the information he's asked for. Don't tell him what to do with the information or he may do the opposite just to let you know who the boss is. Nutty? You bet.

3) While men may talk about independence and autonomy, they are dependent on women much more than you think. Most men appreciate the help you can give them in the areas in which they are least competent. Those areas will probably be anything to do with human relations. Men often have problems with anger, so anything you can do to diffuse a situation or to deal with someone who causes them grief will be appreciated. Men also have problems with clothes, most men, anyway. They appreciate your suggestions and help. A surprising number of men are color blind and need help in a big way. A number of men are just plain lousy at finances and also need help in that important area. If you notice that a man has a problem, offer your help, but don't be too pushy or critical about the way he uses it. Men often need to feel that they're in control.

4) Many men use sports, even in middle age, to handle emotional difficulties. Exercise releases natural tranquilizers into the blood stream called endorphins, which act to calm people under stress. One study we know about says that exercise and diet are about as effective in handling anxiety and depression as drugs and therapy. Men who compulsively run or play sports to the point of hurting themselves do not want to be lectured to. What they want is for someone to understand the reasons they play sports when they're hurt. Lots of men are addicted to exercise. Not to exercise makes them feel worse than doing it when they're hurt. It's called a positive addiction, by the way, because it usually has healthy outcomes.

5) Let men blow off steam, but don't let them blow off steam and expect you to be quiet. You have a right to have a man listen to your feelings as much as he has a right to have you listen to his. The ratio of him listening to you and you to him should be roughly even. If it's out of kilter, let him know. "Hey, Mack. You're hogging the discussion. What about me?" Well, do it a little more sensitively than that, but you get the idea.

6) Don't put men down. It really makes them angry. Don't say anything negative about the sex you're having with your man unless you want to offend him badly. There are gentle and tender ways to discuss sexual problems. Public complaints among friends about how lousy your man is in bed will just make the problem worse. You knew that, I'll bet.

The One Thing All Men Have In Common: The Need for Respect

Men, like everyone else, need to feel that they're respected. When they don't, it makes them a little crazy. Listen to some of my early morning male companions at the coffee shop speak about the way men seem to be treated these days.

Ray, a middle age construction foreman says, "I don't like what's going on. It's always men who get dumped on. Every time some new theory comes out, it's always about how bad men are. There's always some obnoxious psychologist on T.V. going around supporting this stupid theory or that. The minute you hear it, you know it's crap, but everybody goes around repeating it until it's like the truth. When they find out the theory is a bunch of crap, the psychologist isn't anywhere to be found. He or she has made her money over the theory, and so what if a lot of men get screwed because of it."

Jack, a postal supervisor in his early 40's says, "I have a friend whose daughter accused him of raping her. He was shocked. He's got his problems, but that isn't one of them. Turns out the kid is pregnant by some boyfriend who won't admit it and she thinks this is a good way to get out of a jam and make people feel sorry for her. They put my friend through the mill. It nearly killed him. Did anyone come by and say, 'I'm sorry, we made a mistake?' Hell, no. What's a man supposed to believe anymore about the right thing to do? Whatever you do, there's someone around to make you think that you're responsible for everything wrong in the world, just because you're a man."

Raef, a retired railroad switchman says, "I don't think men can be men anymore. It's like everyone wants us to be more like women. If God meant for us to be that way then we'd all be women. I don't see it. I think the country is going to hell because men can't be men anymore. I don't even think women want us to be more like them. I think they want us to be strong and responsible, the way we used to be. When we aren't, that's when they get pissed at us. So many confused boys out there. They don't know about being a man. They learn from the women who raise them and from the streets. How does anyone expect them to know what's right and what isn't?"

Nate, an elderly businessman says, "I think men are the happiest when they're with other men. We can fight and argue and all, but it gets worked out. I don't see a lot of bad men out there. I see a lot of men who feel like crap most of the time because of the way they're treated at work and at home. Most men I know feel their wives and children want the money they bring home but they don't give men the respect they deserve. It can make some of us pretty angry."

Oscar, a plumber in his middle 40's says, "I don't think men have it good anymore. My old man had a position at home. He was respected in the neighborhood. People came to him for advice and help. He was just a good old boy, but he had a nice way with people. Now, everybody thinks that men are rapist and child molesters. No one wants us to spend time with their children out of fear we'll do something awful. We can't be good even if we want to be. My dad just shakes his head when we talk about the world now. He says, 'The psychologists run the show. Those theories of theirs change every week.' All I know is a man can't be a man anymore. I'm glad I'm too old to care.' When I hear that, I get pretty mad. What kind of world is my son going to grow up in? I think I'm doing him wrong by telling him the rules about being a man. It's like training him to be somebody he can't be."

Juan, a retired school teacher who occasionally joins the men at the coffee shop says, "Everybody, including a lot of men, think that men are animals and that we need to be caged up and watched over. I hear male bashing everyday. My wife gets jokes about men that are demeaning. You watch sitcoms and they make men look foolish, like complete imbeciles. And the ads on TV, all about how dumb and one dimensional men are. How does anyone expect that to help young boys grow to be decent men? We let them get away with it. We thought that it wouldn't go so far, and now it has. I don't think we have the ability to do anything about it anymore. It's just like the country. No one knows what to do about anything, so we blame people. Now we blame men. It feels like everything's a little nuts to me. You stand up and defend yourself and everyone looks at you like you're some violent nut case. I never thought that we'd end up being so soft. I was in Nam, for Christ's sake. I killed people I didn't know for this damn country. I spent time in hospitals mending. I still have nightmares about it. And now I'm supposed to believe that the good men around me who died or got maimed, that we're all just rapists and abusers, rapists and abuser? It makes me sick."

You may not agree with any of this. You may feel that men have it a lot better than you do. Maybe they do. Maybe you're right. But you need to understand what many men feel and believe if you want to be able to deal with them. And the reality is that many men feel unappreciated, and to a large extent, they feel they no longer run the show (often, they don't), and it makes them extremely unhappy.

Your job is to understand that many men feel unappreciated. Are they? I don't think so, but compared to the way it used to be when men ran the show, it is different for men. Respect and appreciation are two key words to think about when dealing with most men today. The men who don't deserve either, well, that's another story. But the basically nice guys you know, they deserve to be treated well. Remember: you get more from other people by being nice than by being nasty. That's particularly true for men, but only if they deserve to be treated well.

3

Got No Friends, Never See the Family: Men and Their Relationship Woes

Friends Will Turn On You

My mother used to tell me that a good friend was much better than an uninvolved relative. That isn't the way she said it, of course, but that's the gist of her combination of Yiddish, Polish, English and the soap opera words of wisdom that defined her philosophy of life.

My mother was a lover of soaps. I knew the plots of every soap opera on the radio when I was a kid. When I started telling her what would happen next, however, she stopped telling me the stories. They all, it seemed to my ten year-old mind, had to do with betrayal. Wives to husbands, husbands to wives, siblings to siblings, and, in my mother's mind, and worst of all, friends to friends.

To my mother, a friendship was as sacred as a marriage. This was not a gray area issue for my mother. You had a friend or you didn't. They weren't friends one day and acquaintances the next. A friend was a true and loyal companion who walked through life in your shoes. A friend felt your pain and knew when you were down and needed help. In some mysterious way, according to my mother, they could even read your mind.

Loyalty was everything for my mother. If a friend wasn't loyal, a process not unlike divorce took place. A friend was there when you needed them. You didn't have to spell it out, either. A friend knew when they were needed. When I'd ask how they would know, she'd shrug and say, as millions of Jewish women have said before and since, "don't ask." It was a phrase of wisdom that I could not appreciate until I began to tell my daughter the same thing.

In my mind, a friend is someone who is there for you in your worst moments of crisis. A friend is the person who will take you to the hospital if you are too ill

to go yourself, or to the doctor to hear the possible news of a life threatening illness. A friend can be your husband, or child, or someone very close to you, but
the expectation is the same. You know that when they are needed, a friend will be
there for you, come hell or high water.

Unfortunately, most men almost never expect someone like that to be in their
lives. In fact, men confuse their one or two special friends with the acquaintances
in our lives, the people who come and go but are of little consequence. Most men
disengage from close contact with the people who could be their friends. Much
like love, they don't want to get hurt.

When I was growing up, my father held a view of friendship that was very different from that of my mother. To him, relying on anyone was a terrible mistake.
He'd worked his way from Russia to America as a child, moving slowly across
Europe with his mother and sister, making a few dollars here and there until he
had enough money to come to America. Along the way, he experienced the
depravity and horror of a world gone a little mad after the First World War.

To trust someone, he believed, was a terrible mistake. I don't know that he
trusted his wife or his children. And while he was a remarkable man in many
important ways, he was also a very lonely man who could not share his feelings
and concerns with anyone but me, his oldest son. In his mind, that was my duty
as the oldest son: to protect and defend him, to make sure that nothing bad
would happen to him or to my family. That was why you had a clever son. It
wasn't because he trusted me, or felt close to me, it was more the creation of a
child who would be the caretaker for the family, but especially his caretaker.

When he died, remarkable man that he was, the funeral was empty and deso-
late while my mother's funeral overflowed with people I had never even met. It
was an insight in my life to know the short memory that people had for my
father's many accomplishments.

When my mother died, I can remember walking through a store and listening
to several elderly women talking about her and saying things so sweet and tender
that it was all that I could do not to cry.

My mother knew that you had to give to receive. My father believed that if
you didn't give, then you wouldn't owe anything. My mother's friends were in
the many figures; my fathers were few. When my mother died, the rabbi, who
had never met her said that he'd interviewed her friends and neighbors. She was,
he said, a real Jewish woman: tough, tender and endlessly loyal to her friends and
family. When he said that, I cried for the loss of my mother and for the goodness
she represented in my life. No one would ever be that way for me again, I imag-

ined, for she was my mother, but she was also my friend, and I would miss the loss of both.

Who Will Tie Your Shoes, And Who Will Glove Your Hand?

I tell this story to some ladies I meet for breakfast at the local coffee shop one day and they all nod their heads. They've had husbands and fathers who are friendless. Marjorie, the smart waitress who is just finishing her B.A. in midlife at a university in my community says that it sounds like her husband. "I don't understand it at all," she says. "The man works with more people than you can believe. Everybody likes him, but he isn't close to anyone. Our social life centers around my friends, never his. When I ask him why, he just shrugs his shoulders. I think after twenty years of marriage, he trusts me, sort of. But friends? Forget it. They'll let you down every time. That's what <u>he</u> believes, anyway."

"Why do men have so much trouble making friends?" asks Jana, an older lady who sometimes joins us in the morning, her white hair always neatly done and her fingers twitching for a cigarette now that you can't smoke in restaurants anymore in California. Here's what I tell her.

Men have difficulty finding and making friends because the same thing that makes men fear love, makes them fear friendships. If you get too close to a friend, they'll let you down and you'll get hurt. Men have acquaintances, to be sure, but the one or two real friends who will be there when he really needs one often elude men throughout their lives. The man with real friends is a very lucky person. He knows that his life is rich because of the extension of people who love and care about him, which reminds me of a story I heard several months ago from a fellow passenger on an airline flight.

"I never believed that men needed friends. I grew up with that macho crap that said we men are never ever in need of other people. When my marriage failed several years ago, and I was in shock at how lonely I was, I started to contact my old friends from my old neighborhood. I hadn't seen some of them in twenty years or more. Anyway, I made contact with two guys who were also divorced and lonely. They didn't live where I did, but by calling and seeing them during business trips and the like, we got in touch again.

"They've been a great comfort to me these past several years. I feel closer to them than I ever felt to my wife. We talk, and argue, and drink; men's stuff that I've missed for years. And they're there when I need them. One even came out to visit when I was going through a really bad time of it last year. I don't think there is anyone more lucky than a man who has real friends."

Friend Or Foe: Acquaintances Aren't Friends

Most men confuse friends with acquaintances. An acquaintance is someone we know well, perhaps, but there is no emotional connection between us. We can't expect the same commitment from an acquaintance in time of a crisis that we can from a friend. An acquaintance will move away and we will almost never think of calling to find out how they are. A friend is someone we know and trust in a way similar to that of a spouse or a member of our family.

Men envy women for their many friends, but women are really no different than men. Women generally have many superficial friendships, but few real friends. In our lifetime, we may have a few true friends while we may have unlimited numbers of acquaintances.

As an example of how we confuse friends with acquaintances, I had this discussion over Indian food with the wife of my tennis partner as we all sat eating a meal I was paying for as penance for never bringing tennis balls to our matches:

"In 15 years of marriage," she said, "you're the only friend Jack has ever made. I didn't really think he was capable of friendship, like a lot of men aren't, but you guys have really hit it off."

Now the reality is that I hardly even considered myself an acquaintance. I'd been in Jack's home maybe twice in four years, knew almost nothing about him, and didn't care to know more. For sure, I didn't think of Jack as my friend. But here we were having this strange conversation and it felt to me as if someone I hardly knew was saying that they were in love with me. I thought to myself how different our perceptions were and how interesting it would be to find out why he felt that way since I clearly didn't. So I said, "Yes, playing tennis with Jack allows us to talk about our lives a lot. It's really very nice."

And Jack's wife responded, "Yes, and Jack just never shares information about his life with anyone, not even me." I looked over at Jack and he was beaming. It dawned on me that we all have our standards, our measure of friendship. I had passed Jacks' by listening to him tell a few unrelated and superficial stories about his life. He had failed mine because I found not a shred of evidence that he cared at all about me, or anyone else, and that he was totally self-absorbed.

One day during a tennis match I shared my doctor's concern with him over a medical problem I was having. "You can't live forever," he said. It was a long time before I could play with him and not have an intense feeling of disgust and hostility. And yet, here was a guy who considered me his friend.

It says a whole lot about the way men look at the issue of friendships. So beware when men say that so and so is a friend. From a man's point of view, a friend may be almost anyone who will say good morning to him and not stick a knife in his back. But is that person a true and loyal person who will be there for a man in time of need? More than likely not.

Learn your man's definition of friendship before you believe that anyone is actually a friend. You'd be amazed at how little men know about friendship and how much they confuse a friend with an acquaintance. You can be very helpful to the men in your life by showing them the difference and by helping them form relationships with the men who will be their real friends. You can do this by inviting these men over for dinner or by doing social things together. Sometimes men need guidance in such matters. You'll be surprised how your guidance, if it's not heavy handed, can help men choose friends correctly.

Family: Blood Is Thinner Than Water

Another time, the ladies at the coffee shop ask me about men and their families. Most of the women tell me that their men seem to be continually at war with members of their families. And it's true that family life, for many American men, is often deeply troubled.

When families are healthy, men grow up with positive and affirming messages that help them in their roles as workers, fathers, and husbands. But when men are given unhealthy messages, they grow up holding the confused and distorted beliefs they have learned at home. Men are expected to remain loyal to both healthy and troubled families. Family before anything else. It's a message you hear a lot from the mouths of men who come from troubled families. Be strong, be tough, and be loyal to your family.

When we look at family life, we see a series of alliances between family members. Often these alliances are kept well into adulthood when they seem unhealthy. "Why do we act this way toward one another?" ask the brother and sister or the two brothers who are playing out roles they've learned as children. Because the roles are comfortable and because they've played them so long that they know the roles by heart, that's why.

But of all the interactions that go on among family members, none may be as complex as the interaction between brothers. Brothers are in competition with one another from the beginning. While there may be brothers with deep affection for one another, most of my friends, clients, and colleagues describe their brothers with words like stupid, losers, crazy, eccentric, mean spirited, etc. The fact that their brothers would describe them in exactly the same way seems lost on most of the men I know. For the most part, the conflict between brothers is very great. The ability to resolve differences is so long gone that it seems, for many brothers, to be an impossibility. You listen to men talk about their brothers and after the bluster and the blame, what you mostly hear is sadness. "Why," they seem to be saying, "am I so successful in so many areas of my life and yet so incapable of dealing with someone I should love?"

Maybe the answer is in the way parents taught their male children about the roles they are to play in life. Often those roles are based on birth order. Older brothers are supposed to take care of younger brothers. Younger brothers should worship older brothers. Older brothers are sources of wisdom. Younger brothers should seek older brothers out for knowledge and advice. The more chaotic and dysfunctional the home, the more these messages get played out, often with very bad results.

Two middle-aged brothers I know barely talk to one another even though they live within an hours drive. Whenever they need to talk, they do it by sending sarcastic e-mail messages to each other. When a message goes too far, one stops talking to the other. A year goes by and something happens to bring them together. They court each other like lovers believing that when they get together again, everything will be fine. But when they are together, the anger and the hostility spill over and they both leave, vowing that they will never see one another again.

They have little in common. In many ways, they wouldn't like each other if they were acquaintances. But because they're brothers, part of an immigrant family that stressed loyalty, they play out an increasingly antagonistic game: whatever it takes, this family will stay together. If it doesn't stay together, the family will die, an accurate perception for a Jewish family whose relatives mostly perished in the Holocaust and are now few in number.

The older brother confides in me. He is my friend. I listen to his angry outbursts at his brother, many of which seem unjust. What I feel is how very sad my friend is whenever his brother is mentioned. It feels to me as if he's in mourning for a dead brother.

"It must be difficult to constantly resurrect a dead brother just to please your parents," I tell him, sure that he will take offense.

"I do, don't I," he says. "I really don't like the offensive little shmuck (jerk). I can only see him at his house. He won't come to mine now that he's so religious.

This is a brother I've bailed out of jail for drug possession, who I repeatedly helped when he was younger because my folks thought I had responsibility for him. I go to his house now and watch this charade with the religious stuff, and I'm immensely offended. He treats me and my sister like we were idiots, worms. I want to punch him out. It's all I can do to stay and not say something that will upset everyone there.

"If it weren't for this feeling I still have of loyalty to the family, I'd forget him and move on in my life. He's certainly not a factor anymore, he's just an irritant. I know we have a sick relationship. I suspect that he knows it, as well. It's just that I feel stuck in this role I've always played as the older brother who saves his hide when he's in trouble. Well, he's not in trouble anymore and what he does to thank me for helping him in the past is to ridicule me."

Another set of brothers I know have such long forgotten animosities between them that they no longer remember the reasons for their anger. The younger brother complains that the older one is such a know-it-all that it makes him angry to even be near him. The older brother accuses the younger one of torpedoing the relationship with his constant attacks on the brother's intelligence. One is college trained while the other put his brother through college at the price of being denied his own education. The older brother complains that he's never been thanked for the help he gave. The younger one says that a day doesn't go by that the older brother hasn't demanded that he acknowledge the help he gave.

And so it goes. Each encounter between them is a set of subtle put downs. Last year, the two came to blows at a party. Their children had to separate them. Both went away without apologizing to the other. I was called in to help mediate between them. It was impossible. The room where we met to discuss the situation was so filled with anger that you could cut it with a knife.

"You ungrateful shit," the older brother screamed out before we had even begun.

"You ignorant piece of crap," yelled the younger brother.

"I should have let you go to college on your own, you lazy bastard."

"You did let me go alone. You threw a few bucks at me and demanded that I worship the ground you walk on. I wouldn't worship anything about you, you shit."

Finally, I stepped in and asked them why they were so angry at one another. As it turned out, it wasn't the college thing, it was something else. They looked stupefied. Nothing. They couldn't think of anything. Well, maybe there was something, thought the older brother. "Maybe," he said, "maybe it's all about the way dad used to make me take care of you. He said that you were the smart one and I was the strong one. That you needed my help, but that I was able to take care of myself."

The younger brother looked confused. "I don't know what you're talking about," he said.

"No, of course. It happened when we were very young. I was maybe seven and you were two, but he'd already decided that I wasn't bright enough. I mean, how the hell do you think that made me feel? How did he know that I wasn't bright? What nerve he had doing that. And the worst part was that I believed him. I didn't think I was smart enough for college, and how I resented you. I hated you with a passion."

They both looked at each another. Grown men still playing out roles assigned to them as children. Still bitter and hateful over the inequities of their father's behavior, neither responsible for what had happened, and both of them suffering the consequences of the terrible mistakes a parent had make.

They left the meeting still angry, still overwhelmed with resentment. Old animosities die hard. More is the shame for the millions of brothers at war with each other over the mistakes of their parents.

The Sorry Times of Family Life

Many of the people I talk to are angry at their families. Blood doesn't guarantee love. A family is like a small organization with conflicting loyalties. We use the term "dysfunctional" to describe the families who were troubled when men were growing up. It might be more helpful to describe those families as having very different ideas about how best to do the job of surviving.

A troubled family may use put downs or corporal punishment to instill toughness. It may deny love to prepare people for life as parents see life. A troubled family may turn child against child or play favorites among the children to make children more competitive. I'm not saying this as a positive, mind you, but as an explanation of the reason troubled families act the way they do. The outcome, of course, is that children raised in troubled families have difficulty getting along with each other. And often, that difficulty may be carried over into their personal lives. The abused child becomes the abusive parent. The unloved son becomes the unloving husband. The emotionally abused daughter becomes the abused girlfriend and wife.

The amazing thing in troubled families is how each member of the family views the trouble from a very different perspective. An ex-client, as these dialogues will show, sees his mother as an ogre while the elderly mother can't understand his current animosity toward her.

The Son: "When I was growing up, my mother and father were so enmeshed with one another that we kids pretty much felt like the hired help. When my dad died, my mom had secret alliances with all of the kids, which bordered on the perverse. Everything was slightly sexualized. She'd let us see her naked. She'd always wear sexy clothing around the house. I hated being around her. I thought she was this childish, immature old hag who ignored us when my dad was around and was now trying to seduce us. I saw our home as being immensely unhappy. I couldn't wait to leave it, I hated it so much. And I hated her the most. My brothers and sisters and I keep some sort of peace. We manage, in a hollow way, to get along. But no one gets along with my mother. She's past 70 and she's still trying to seduce us. And hating her the most, guess who's stuck with caring for her? Me."

The Mother: "When my husband died, it was very difficult. I had 4 small kids. I was tired from working all of the time. I didn't go out with men because I thought it would upset the kids and, anyway, I was too tired from working all day. The kids were difficult after George died. They wouldn't mind me at all. I wondered if they thought that I was to blame for George's death. Kids have a funny way of seeing things, I guess. I went to a counselor to get help, I even took the kids in a few times, but they complained about it so much that I stopped. I did the best I could, but the kids never helped out the way I needed them to. Now I'm staying with my son Johnny. He's so nasty to me it's worse than being in a nursing home. I ask to leave and then he becomes apologetic, and I stay. I have no idea why they're all so hateful. George and I were good parents. After he died, I tried hard to be a good parent. You can only do so much for kids, I guess."

Troubled Memories Of Family Life

While I was writing this chapter on friends and family, I asked my graduate social work class to describe any problems they were having with family. Of 25 students, every student was experiencing problems. Many of the men in the class had not spoken to brothers in years. One woman said that she'd not spoken to her mother since 1989 when, at the funeral of her son who had died in a car crash, her mother said, "You've got three other children, a husband, and plenty of money. But look at me. I'm alone and poor, and nobody cares about me anymore."

Another woman in my class said that she'd not spoken to her brothers and sisters in 15 years until the thought of growing old by herself drove her closer to her siblings. They still have, she said, an "uneasy" relationship. Another student said that of the 3 brothers he has, none has spoken to the other in more than 10 years and that even after their father died, they refused to speak to one another at the funeral.

This is the condition of family life for all too many American men and women. Listen to another example of American family life from one of my graduate students in a workshop I recently taught.

"My family was so screwy that when I think about it, I shudder."

"What was so wrong?" I asked.

"It was a group of strangers living under the same roof. No one had anything in common. I used to think that my brother was illegitimate and that my sister was adopted. I still think that, as a matter of fact. Whenever I see them, I know that they aren't my real siblings. I mean, my brother is a cop, for Chrissake."

"What's wrong with that?" I asked, now really confused.

"He hates Blacks and Hispanics. He loves guns, worships them, belongs to the NRA. Underneath it all, he's probably a white supremacist. Every time we talk, we almost come to blows. And my sister, my sister's a goddamn 'right to lifer.' She's out on the picket lines against abortions. Where did these people come from? They have nothing in common with me."

"But what about them as people?" I asked. "Are they O.K. people?"

He shrugged and looked away for a while. "Yeah, I guess you could say that. They're O.K. people."

"Then why the animosity? I don't see the reason?"

He thought for a while, shook his head, and looked at his feet. "I just don't think they're very thoughtful or sensitive people. They aren't people I care to be around."

I asked him about blood being thicker than water and wasn't that more important than whether he liked his family.

"They're ignorant people," he said. "I can't see wasting my time with them. Anyway, I don't buy this loyalty to family stuff. I don't think families' do much more than shelter and feed you until you're on your own. Maybe they used to, but not anymore. My dad could hardly wait to kick me out when I was 18. What loyalty should I have? I've been on my own most of my life. I asked for little, and that's pretty much what they gave me. People get mushy about families, but as far as I'm concerned, they're a crock. We could do better with orphanages and Kibbutz's. Families molest, and abuse, and fail to nurture. I think they're outdated. I know that's a sacrilege, but it's how I feel. I'll bet a lot of people feel that way."

The women at the coffee shop cluck when they hear this last story. "It's shameful to feel that way about your family," one of them says. Another says, "There must be something wrong with that young man. No wonder he's in social work. He's trying to work his problems out, I'll bet." No one wants to hear what a mess our families are in, but after a few minutes, the ladies begin to share similar stories. Their families aren't so red hot either, they tell us, but they thought it was just <u>their</u> family and not everyone else's. They sit for a while in gloomy silence reliving past and present hurts so deep that you can see a look of sorrow in everyone's eyes, including mine.

You want family to be there for you. You want to believe in the goodness of family life. It's reassuring to think that someone will be out there when the cruelties of life push in on you. How fortunate are the men and women with helpful, caring families.

Why Families Don't Always Work

I'm asked one morning to explain why there are such bad feelings between family members that continue on into adulthood? It isn't an easy question because there are so many reasons and many of them, such as poverty and loss of jobs, are out of the control of family members. But these are the reasons I gave the ladies at the coffee shop:

1) Because of unresolved feelings in childhood. The hurts and slights experienced in childhood have a way of adding up, particularly when men are involved. Men seldom work these feelings of anger at family through. Instead, they keep angry feelings inside where they fester, and grow, and increase with every hurtful encounter with a family member.

2) Because the closeness of family life, like marriage, offers many opportunities for hurt feelings and difficulties across the entire span of life.

3) Because some of us were raised in dysfunctional homes where petty jealousies were intensified into major problems.

4) Because some of us experienced physical and emotional abuse at the hands of a family member and it doesn't easily go away from our view of that person or of the family experience.

5) Because we are in competition with our brothers and sisters for the love and affection of our parents. Even after our parent's die, that behavior often continues.

6) Because we change and we may not like the adult version of some of our family members.

7) Because adulthood is a time of considerable envy, and siblings may have exceeded us in their lives.

8) Because, as adults, we have different views of life that may be out of synch with those of family members. This may be true of religious and political beliefs and the way we live our lives, raise our children, believe in education, etc. People change, even the people we grew up with.

And The Ladies Have The Last Word

"Boy, doc, you sure are hard on families, you know?" It's Emalinda talking, a transplanted New Yorker by way of Puerto Rico. "I think families do some terrific things for kids. Sure they screw up sometimes, but they're the best thing we got going."

Linda, a new mom with two young children, agrees. "My family didn't do such a good job," she says, "but I still love them. They tried as hard as they could and they did a good job, considering all the problems we had including my dad being laid off his job and my mom being sick. We all worked together at my house and we still work together."

Gina, a new high school graduate learning the ropes on a new job chimes in, "I think my brothers had it better than me and my sister. They weren't expected to do anything around the house while me and my sisters were treated like slaves."

Edna, a woman in her early sixties who sits with us silently with a bemused look on her face adds, "Doc, men have it so much better than women in families. They don't have to cook, or clean, or do much of anything. Everybody kowtows to them and treats them special. My boy's think they're gods while they think they're sisters should wait on them and take care of their needs. I think men have it pretty good in families when they're growing up."

The consensus around the table is that men have it made while women are treated like dirt in most families. Personally, I think that lots of children are treated badly, boys and girls, but that's another story for another time.

We file out of the coffee shop on our way to work. Crystal stretches the remaining sleep out of her body before jumping into her truck. We both stand and watch the sun come up over the mountains and Crystal says, "It's gonna be a pretty one, doc. No one can take that away from us," and she drives off into the rising sun, waiving at me while my heart flutters.

4

Pretty Woman: Love Can Drive Men Crazy

The War Zone: Men in Love

Most of the women I talk to can't understand why men act the way they do when they're in love. It all seems pretty illogical to them. One minute the man they're in love with is writing them corny poetry and sending roses, and the next minute, they're sarcastic and distant.

I try to explain to them that when men are in love, they get a little crazy. It's a craziness that never ceases to amaze women. In the midst of this craziness, men lose control of their emotions. They feel wonderful and awful at the same time. The wonder of love makes men, even hardened men, feel warmth and caring so deep inside that, for many men, it's a new and incredibly painful experience.

Love unleashes strong feelings of jealousy and men often start to have obsessive thoughts that lovers are unfaithful to them. Men also believe that there are hidden reasons a women is seeing them, reasons other than the obvious one that a women likes, respects, admires, feels right, and even, praise the heavens, might be in love with them. And I mean all men go through this period of anxiety, even bright and educated men who ought to know better, who do know better, in fact.

When the jealousy they experience begins to overwhelm them, men distance themselves from their women. They may say hurtful and sarcastic things to their women. Women are dismayed when this happens. Correctly, they haven't a clue as to why their lovers suddenly turn on them.

The fact is that men are frightened by love. It's an emotion with which they have little experience. In it's grip, they feel as vulnerable as children. Just as they can't love their wives and girlfriends, often they can't love their children because children might turn on them. Since men have often turned on their parents, it makes sense to them that they must distance themselves from their children before something awful happens. The awful thing that might happen is that they will love their children and not have that love returned.

For many men, the need for love and intimacy and the fear of love and intimacy are conflicting emotions that play themselves out as men age. Increasingly, fear of intimacy is the emotion that wins out. But not without a terrible price. That price is loneliness and a growing sense of isolation from people. And because loneliness is everything it's cracked up to be, men suffer when they're lonely. They drink too much and become strange in their personal habits. Without women to guide them and to keep them in touch with the world around them, many men float away into a sort of cosmic exile where television and drink are their addictions and jobs are their only contact with people.

Some men learn to have sex with women for whom they feel nothing. This arrangement is a perfect prescription for impotence and other sexual problems. Some men marry or have relationships and feel dead inside. They play-act or feign affection but inside, where the heart is, they are emotionless and distant. For many men, this unwillingness to feel anything for another human being leads to depression, sleep disorders, and alcohol and drug use as a way of dealing with the emptiness they feel inside.

My good friend Marjorie Callaghan, who knows a lot about men and women, tells me that many older men have turned away from women. Hurt, once too often, they live their lives free of entanglements just as many older women do the very same thing. Fear of being hurt is a universal concern among the solitary warriors in the sex wars.

Women often think that men are too self-centered or cold to love them. But the truth is that men believe that they feel too strongly. If women knew how vulnerable they were, men believe, then women would take advantage of them. And since men have been taught to believe that women are capable of sucking the marrow from their bones, being taken advantage of can lead to the worst kind of sorrow.

For many men, reassurance, even if it seems unnecessary, is a way to get men to commit. For other men, time and consistency help men feel more comfortable with love. But for some men, nothing helps. The harm they inflict on themselves and on others in the process of protecting themselves from being hurt is so destructive, that they and their loved ones often never completely recover. These are the men who are loving and tender one minute and then abandon wives and children the next.

Fear of rejection often propels men to do the dismal and hurtful things they sometimes do to women; out of spite, out of fear, out of the primitive need men have to defend their pride. The behavior of many men in love drives women crazy. It just doesn't make sense to them.

Fear and Loathing in the Bedroom

It should come as no surprise that men often confuse sex with love. Not knowing how to be intimate and fearing love, they assume that sex is the same as love. Maybe it helps to explain the jealous rages men go into after they've had sex with a woman. The woman may be disappointed that sex hasn't lead to greater intimacy but from the man's point of view, sex <u>is</u> intimacy.

Men often chase women for whom they feel little affection just to successfully have sex with them. This conquest, which ends in sex, allows a man to have bragging rights since he can now think of himself as sexual, romantic, and virile while the woman he chased so hard thinks that it's actually love he's showing her; love, and affection, and the desire for intimacy. Of course, this isn't true of all men and many men share these emotions with someone they care about.

One of my colleagues, in the midst of this behavior, came to a party of mine with his newest love interest. He was solicitous, charming, gallant, and every few minutes, he held the lady and said romantic things in her ear. Looking on, the wife of a friend turned to me and said, "That's Ethan's imitation of Macho Man, you know. He comes on like gang busters, chases the woman all over the place, and gives her more than any man in the history of the world has ever given a woman. Then he gets bored. Women can't understand it. They think he's so wonderful and then he drops them cold. All he cares about is the chase."

After four wives and a playing field strewn with shattered, angry women, many of whom have called me wondering how I can be his friend when he's such a jerk, it's hard to understand why he hasn't changed. He knows enough to get women to adore him, but he knows almost nothing about sustaining a relationship. Instead of learning about women and committing himself to a long-term relationship, he fills the relationship with sex, adoration, and endless activity, and then he moves on to his next conquest.

I've tried to talk to him about his behavior, but he thinks he knows a whole lot more about women than I do. His behavior is called Don Juanism, after the famous lover, Don Juan. To change his behavior, Ethan would have to understand that he just doesn't like or respect women.

For whatever reason, men who chase women and then drop them when the chase is over have a great deal of anger at women. Maybe it stems from problems in the early relationship with mothers, or maybe it's because men have been rejected by women early in life. Whatever the cause, men like Ethan, while charming and exciting, can do major harm to women. For this reason, stay away from Don Juan's, ladies, they're killers.

Men Who Think Women Like Bad Boys

Some men believe that women want their men to be very bad. In high school it seemed to many young men that the guys who treated their women badly were the guys girls loved to be with. Because of this, many adult men believe that being nice to a woman doesn't have much payoff. Listen to a friend of mine talk about the mistakes he made in his last marriage:

"I stuck it out for 11 years with my last wife. I would like to have everyone of them back, that's how little I got out of our marriage. She thought that my job in life was to make her happy. And because she was never happy, she came to think that it was my fault. I was so screwed up most of the time that I started to agree with her. She's living with some guy who abuses her and she loves him, adores him. It makes me feel like an idiot for putting all of that time into being nice when there was more payoff for being abusive."

It's acceptable to some men to run from a relationship when it gets to be too demanding because women, they believe, will enjoy this act of defiance. This should help explain the numerous men who abandon wives, girlfriends, and families and who believe that such behavior endears them to others rather than hurting them beyond repair.

Consider another story of a colleague who practices bad boy behavior and abandonment. "My wife and I never did anything," my colleague told me. "It was like living with a relative or kissing your sister. We had a child together and a nice house, but we were never connected by love or passion. All she did was criticize me. Continually. Nothing I did was good enough. One day I just had enough and left. I deserve better than that after all of these years of working so hard and Isabella (his long-time girl friend) and I can have something together that Jean and I never had."

Three months after leaving his wife for Isabella, I came home from a long trip to find him camping out at my house, his bags and boxes scattered all over my garage. "What happened?" I asked.

"I don't know. All Isabella wanted to do was to criticize me. It was like being with my wife, only the sex was better. I couldn't work, I couldn't think, I was in turmoil all the time. I asked my wife to take me back. She's not happy about it but I think she will." The next night Isabella called me up to talk.

"I can't understand it," she said. "I thought we were doing so well. I thought he was so happy. He seemed to be. And then one night we got into an argument and the next thing I know, he's left without even giving me a reason. He didn't even say goodbye. Have I missed something?" she asked.

I wondered how well I knew my friend. He seemed alright to me, but then I wasn't living with him. I talked to him a few days later. "I came home from work late," he told me "and she'd (Isabella) made a bed up for me in the spare bedroom, punishment for some imaginary thing I'd done to her. When I asked her the next morning what I'd done, she couldn't believe that I wasn't aware of how angry she was at me. I'd like some peace in my life, you know? I'm not a mind reader. Women are so damn vague. It drives me nuts."

"Couldn't you have talked it out?" I asked. "Isabella seems like a pretty wise person."

"I tried, but the more we talked, the madder I got. Why should I have to explain myself all of the time to women? Shit, they don't explain themselves to me. And anyway, why put energy into being nice to them? You can treat them like crap and they'll always take you back. I treated Jean badly for twenty years. I had affairs and spent weeks away from the house without calling her, and she's always taken me back. Isabella will do the same. You'll see."

In my earlier conversation with Isabella, she'd said, "You know, he never paid for anything. He left wet towels on the bed and tracked dirt all over the house. He didn't pay for the rent or for any food. Of <u>course</u> I nagged him about it. Who wouldn't? What kind of way is that to treat me, especially from someone who says they love me? I'm trying to understand his behavior and, I confess, I can't. He left his wife and says that I put pressure on him to come live with me when I didn't. Then, because of a couple of minor arguments, he leaves me to return to a wife he divorced who he says he hates. He thinks he can treat women like dirt and we'll always be there for him, but he's wrong. Some of us won't put up with it."

At the core of my friend's behavior are three typically male beliefs. One, my friend believes that once a women is in love with a man, no matter how badly he treats her, she'll love him forever. Two, hurtful behavior such as abandonment actually increases the love a woman has for a man. And three, that criticism by a woman is an act which is meant to rob men of their manliness. Remember that even Freud had a term for critical women. He called them "castrating."

In my friend's mind, leaving women was completely acceptable. Having little regard for women to begin with, he believed that walking away from a relationship would force the woman to change her behavior. And having acted badly, he was convinced that his behavior would actually endear him to women. Long after he'd stopped seeing Isabella, in fact, he tried to start the relationship up again.

"He came to the house and stayed in the driveway all night long," she told me later. "He'd been drinking heavily. He was screaming at me, calling me ungrateful and other names I won't mention. He thought he had the right to see me again just because...well, just because he had the right. I can't understand how anyone would think that way. He still calls me and writes letters as if he hasn't acted like the worlds biggest jerk. I blame myself. I thought he was such a smart and successful man that he'd never act that way, but I guess the smarter they are, the more they think women will fall for their bad boy routines. It just isn't so."

Bad boys do hurtful things. They believe that women enjoy their bad behavior. And contrary to what age and experience tells them, many men continue to mistreat women when they're in love because they believe it will only make women love them more. It's a bit of craziness that takes a little time to comprehend. The best way to understand bad boy behavior is to recognize that while high school may be well behind them, for too many men, it's their major introduction to the art and science of loving someone. They continue to believe that what worked in high school will work forever.

Lies Men Tell Each Other About Women

How fragile can a man's ego be when men are out in the world of work everyday fighting to stay on top of the competition? And the answer is that when it comes to love and intimacy, the ego of most men is as fragile and as a delicate as a piece of china.

Men are, for lack of a better way of putting it, prisoners to the lies they tell each other about women. Rather than viewing women as individuals and respecting the uniqueness of a single woman, men often believe the assorted myths and stories they hear about women while growing up. In time, these stories become the wisdom of the male species as it relates to women. That these stories are often hopelessly inaccurate should help give women an idea of how troubled men in love can be. Let's consider some of the mistaken ideas that men in love have about women.

I. Whore or Saint?

Men often believe that women are pure, chaste and saintly. At the same time, they often approach women as if they're easy prey for sexual advances. This confusion about women forces men to put women into two separate camps. In the first camp is every woman who ever fell hook, line, and sinker for a series of lies meant only to get them in bed. In the other camp are those women a man truly loves and respects. Mothers, sisters, wives, and daughters fall into this later camp. The problem for men is how to confer saintliness on the same women they previously considered to be tramps since their wives and girlfriends often come from that sector of the sexually active universe they reserve for most women.

To accommodate this confusion over the purity of the women they love, men want to believe that women have never had sex with anyone else, have never been truly in love with another man, have never had an orgasm before having sex with them, never think about other men, and are absolutely sexless in their preoccupations with life except for the sexual feelings they have for their specific man. This, as all too many women who have been grilled by lovers or husbands about their past love lives, is the saint part of equation.

This absurd way of looking at women gets men into a great deal of difficulty. For one thing, it leads to obsessive jealousy. How, a man wonders irrationally, could this woman I love so much have gone to bed with someone else? Because they slept with another man or many other men, does that make her the whore I believe most women actually are? And if she's a whore, should I love her? Won't awful things happen to me if I fall in love with someone who might be unfaithful to me in the long run?

This need to make all women they love into saints can drive insecure men a little crazy with jealousy, as this story from a former female client should demonstrate.

"My boyfriend John and I were out for a drink when we met an old flame of mine. John was very pleasant to my ex, but you could tell that he was seething underneath it all. When we got home, he started to grill me about Ted. Was he any good in bed? Did I enjoy sex with him? Did I ever think about him or call him up? And finally, was I seeing him now? Why, he kept on asking, did Ted show up in a bar in a large city like Los Angeles since he supposedly lived many miles away?

"I told him that I hadn't thought about Ted in a long time and that I was so in love with him (John, my current boyfriend) that I never thought about anyone but him. And I lied about my relationship with Ted, which had been wonderful while it lasted, because John was so upset that I could feel his body shaking and hear his voice quivering as he asked me these questions.

"I don't know about men. Why are they so insecure about women? They go out and do the craziest things, things that are dangerous and nutty and risky, but when it comes to women, they're so insecure and childlike that you can't believe it's the same person. I think men should be given a course in understanding women so they don't all act like asses when they're in love.

"This is the fourth or fifth guy I've gone with who ended up grilling me about former boyfriends. But you ought to listen to them brag about their sexual exploits. Boy, talk about a double standard. Women are supposed to be perfect and never sleep with a man until they're married, and if they did, then they're not supposed to have enjoyed it much. But men can brag all they want to and the woman is supposed to admire the guy for being such a stud. It really tells me how insecure guys are when it comes to love."

The thought of a woman they love being with another man drives most men a little crazy. I remember a felon I interviewed in jail, a very bad human being who had done terrible things to people, cry while telling me that he'd found his wife with another man. He had arms like tree stumps and he was crying. He'd been a mean and abusive man to all the women he'd known, but he kept asking how someone could do something so mean to him. "Women," he said, finally, "you can't trust them and you can't believe in them. They'll kill you if you do."

Why had he treated his women so badly? And having treated his women so badly, why not be a bit more accepting about what happened? Because, as he explained to me, "You love a woman. You give her everything you can. Sometimes you don't act good, and sometimes you stray, but a woman has to stay faithful or you got nothing else to believe in this world." And he, like most men, absolutely believed that to the core of his being.

II. Women Will Be By Your Side Come Hell or High Water

Another lie. Women are the glue that keeps this crazy world together. A man can stray and act badly, but women will always be around to pick up the pieces. This bit of mythology is actually one that women rather like to tell about themselves so it has more clout with men than other lies men tell about women. The fact is, however, that men use this myth to justify a great deal of bad behavior and then reinforce that bad conduct by believing that women will always be there to take care of their mistakes, so why not act badly?

I've heard this same attitude used to justify just about every piece of terrible male behavior imaginable from abandoning children, to drinking too much, to abusing children, girlfriends, and wives. You can endlessly mistreat a woman and they'll stay by your side in sickness, in bad health, and in misery.

Superwoman. You touch a man deep down inside and they'll tell you that women have super powers. Part of this mythology about women is based on the way mothers were in the face of considerable odds. "My mom was a saint," the hardened criminal will tell you and his eyes will become misty. Underneath every man's notion of womanhood is the belief that women have super powers and that their saintliness will never permit them to do anything in retribution for a man's bad conduct. This is another lie that lets men treat the women they love very badly.

III. Women Are Slaves To Men

Men believe that women are slaves to their needs. Those needs may be sexual or the everyday needs men have in their lives. But deep down inside, most men think that women are subservient and that men have a right to ask of them just about anything they want. When a man is in love, that can be quite a lot, as this story from a former female client will show.

"I was seeing Larry, a middle aged guy who worked in my store. He was a nice enough person but whenever we were together, he'd sit around and wait for me to serve him. He never offered to help around the house. When we'd have dinner at my house, he'd sit around watching T.V. while I cooked and did the dishes. It was annoying to me so I asked him for some help. You know what he said? He said that men who help around the house are sissies. Worse, he said that any man who didn't know that women were supposed to do the work around the house was a man women would step all over.

"Well, I stepped all over him all right. I told him in no uncertain terms that either he helped a little or he could just walk right out of my life. And you know what? He got up and walked out of the house. I can't believe in this day and age that any man would be so narrow minded, but when I talk to other women, they tell me the same thing. Where do men learn such nonsense? Does every man's mother treat him like a child all of his life? I have boys and they know how to help around the house. I don't know, maybe it's our fault for letting guys act like we're slaves."

IV. The Psychic Healer

Finally, it seems to me that men expect women to come rushing to them with apologies, to read their minds when they hurt, to know instinctively when they're in need. Reading minds is a requisite skill all women are supposed to have and the lies men tell about women set impossibly high standards for female sensitivity.

"You are supposed to know that I expect you to call when I come back from a trip," says the tired male executive to his lover.

"What rule says that you can't call me?" responds the woman.

"I'm tired and lonely after a trip," comes the reply. "You ought to know that, and if you were sensitive to my needs, you'd call."

"But you don't call me when I return from a trip."

"It's not the man's place to call, it's the woman's."

"Where is that written? I've never heard such hog wash."

"If you were a sensitive and loving woman instead of being competitive and cold, you'd know that."

And on and on it goes. Such is the way that men sometimes think about women. From a man's point of view, women are supposed to know the crazy social rules they think guide relationships. And if they don't know the rules, should the man explain them? Of course not. The man's job is to criticize the woman for breaking rules she never knew existed in the first place. Crazy? You bet.

And The Ladies Have The Last Word

These bits and pieces of wisdom about men have been shared with the men and women of the coffee shop over months of discussion. As always, the women sit and stare at me as I discuss men, disbelieving what I've said at first, and then seeing the men nod their heads in agreement, they become resigned to the fact that men in love can be a handful and a half.

Laura, a young, newly widowed woman looks at me after a particularly troubling discussion of how men expect women to be psychic mind readers. "You know," she says, "I never told anyone this while I was married, but after my husband started getting sick and I was urging him to go to see a doctor, he actually blamed me for his illness. He said that I should have seen the problem coming and I should have called the doctor and asked him what to do. When it turned out that he had a terminal illness, he stopped talking to me. He thought it was my fault. If I'd acted earlier, he kept saying, he'd be O.K. now.

"I loved my husband and I know he was sick and all, but where do men get such ideas? Where did he get off blaming me for his illness? I feel guilty to this day that I did something to make him sick and then didn't take care of him. I know it sounds nutty, but that's the way it was left when he died."

Everybody sits and looks off in space. Finally, one of the women says to the group, "I think we have a lot of work to do with our sons. I can see now that I should have taken the time to teach them about women. I thought they'd learn from experience, but from what doc says and from what we all know, they don't learn much at all. It's time we taught them that women are human beings, not saints or superwomen."

Everyone applauds except one of the men who sits in a corner with a troubled look on his face. Before we breakup and move on to our jobs he says, "Men bring home the food and we protect the women and children. Women raise the kids. God made us different so we could have families. That's the way it's supposed to be."

To which one of the women in the group replies, "Bull shit! You've learned nothing at all, mister, not a thing. Go back to the corner and sit with the men who still think beating a woman is good for her mental health."

And you know what? He did.

5

The Intelligent Woman's Guide to Men in Love: Good Luck, You'll Need It!

Sex Wars: The Rules of Engagement

It's early in the morning and I'm sitting with some ladies at the coffee shop, shooting the breeze. "What do they want from us?" Crystal, an attractive woman in her mid-forties asks. "I've been around the block a few times (everybody at the table nods appreciatively) and I don't know much more about men and love than I did when I was a teen-ager."

Angie, another one of the regulars I see most mornings at the coffee shop says, "Me too. The older I get, the more I think men are off in some crazy world of their own and what they think about women is nuts. How can you love a crazy man? That's the way they act when they're in love, I swear."

Everyone around the table agrees that when men are in love, look out Nellie! it's time to can the peaches and prepare for a long, hard winter.

Over the years, I've come to believe that there are a few serious mistakes that women make when moving from liking a man to loving him. It seems to me that not making these mistakes will level the field enough to make the crazy process of dealing with the men you love a little easier. And remember that I said a <u>little</u> easier. It's never easy to deal with men in love, so prepare yourself for the rocky road ahead because never, in the history of the world has it been easy to love a man and expect him to act in a sane and predictable way. So here goes, ladies. Here are the rules of engagement when dealing with the man you love.

Rule 1: Make A Man Jealous And There's Hell To Pay

Don't make men jealous. If you think that getting back at a man for something he's done by making him jealous is a good idea, it' not. There's hell to pay for that sort of thinking. Jealousy is a losing emotion. It can't possibly lead to anything good. Listen to what one man I know thought about a relationship he had and then imagine how jealous most men are and the terrible things that can happen in a relationship.

"I had absolutely no reason to believe that Linda was being unfaithful to me. None. And yet I knew in my heart that she was having sex with every man who walked. It drove me nuts. A smile at the wrong moment, a look on her face, a letter she didn't share with me, and I knew she was with someone else, everyone else, every man in the world. This is someone who wouldn't go to bed with me before we were married for what seemed like a lifetime. This is someone who was really hurt in a bad marriage. This is the most loving and tender woman I've ever known and I blew it to hell by these jealous rages I'd go into. Where the hell they came from, I'll never know.

"Linda was appalled. She's a refined woman. Hell, <u>I'm</u> a refined guy, and here I am accusing her of screwing the entire UCLA Football Team, or something like that. It was madness. Finally, we sat down and talked it out. She assured me that I was the only one in her life and that she couldn't possibly sleep with anyone else. We tried to get at the root of what was going on. I'd never been in love before. <u>Really</u> been in love. It was a new experience for me. In other relationships, a part of me stayed aloof from the woman for fear of getting hurt. With Linda, it all hung out and I loved her with everything inside of me.

"Thank God we talked because I gradually came to trust her and we're married now. She's such a wonderful woman, I almost blew it with jealousy. It's a terrible emotion to deal with. It consumes you, it really does. It doesn't take anything for men to be jealous. I know of women who intentionally make men jealous. It's a big mistake. When I was at the height of my jealous feelings, I came very close to physically hurting a woman I love very much. If any woman thinks it'll make men commit to them by playing one guy off against another, it won't. If anything, it's likely to destroy a relationship."

Get the picture? Men are very suspicious when they're in love. They can't understand why this wonderful woman, you, is so nice to them. They don't think they deserve to be treated so well. They think if they're in love, it makes them weaker and they fight the feeling like crazy. Just don't give them a chance to fight love. Be calm, honest, tender, and loving. Be consistent. Inconsistency is a sure sign to men that something is wrong.

If you're not feeling well but you can still manage a date, do it. Let the man see that you think enough of him to see him even if you aren't well. Don't talk about other love or dating experiences with men. It makes men very angry and don't let him talk about other experiences with women, either. It'll make <u>you</u> nuts. Approach men with all of the sensitivity and tenderness you have inside. Believe me, you'll hook men in no time just by being considerate. Most men pay hell during the day at work. A little tenderness can go a very long way in a man's life.

Rule 2: The Way A Man Was With Other Women Will Tell You How He'll Be With You

The way a man has acted in the past with women will often tell you how he's going to act with you. If he's had problems with women before, don't think that you're so special that the same thing won't happen to you. When a man implies that he has skeletons in his closet, believe him. Do not…listen to me now…do not believe that you will be the great love who will change his ways. It's a fantasy which has driven more than a few women to great anguish and sorrow. Consider this story from one of my former female clients.

"I guess I have broken wing syndrome. I must believe that I can make the sick well and the crazy, sane. I started seeing Joe. He was up front with me, I'll say that about him. He told me that he had serious psychological problems, that he slept around and had never been able to love one woman exclusively. It just made me love him more.

"He was my project, my mission in life. When I was done with him, he'd be rehabilitated. He'd never want to sleep with anyone else in the world except me. And did I treat that man well. He never had it so good. And then I'd see this far away look in his eyes and I should have known that he was thinking about someone else. But no, social worker that I was, I took it for love. This went on for months.

"He was starting to miss dates and not return my calls. It made me work all the harder. Finally, I saw him out with some really slutty looking woman. She was hanging all over him. I went a little crazy and confronted him. He listened to me for a while and then he took me aside and said that he couldn't stand the sight of me and to get out of his life, that he was sick of me being so nice to him all the time. He wasn't a nice person and he resented being treated so well. And that was that.

"It's broken wing syndrome in women. We think we can fix damaged men. We look for them, find them, and try and make them well. And then, predictably, we get hurt. I look at someone now and try and find out about their past. If it's screwy, if they've had lots of problems, I run like crazy. My broken wing syndrome is gone. Find someone healthy. It's tough enough with a good man. With a sick one, it's impossible."

Rule 3: You Can't Make A Man Love You If He Won't

Don't think that you can make a man love you if the evidence, all of it, suggests that he doesn't. Men don't grow slowly into love. Like you, they start to feel infatuation fairly early on in a relationship. But if he clearly hasn't moved into infatuation, and if you see absolutely no evidence that he will ever love you, then accept the truth and move on. Certainly, it always hurts when someone we love doesn't love us back, but it's an early hurt and it's easier to get over than the hurt that lingers when you stay indefinitely in a relationship with a man who does not, and will not, love you.

A student of mine told me a troubling story about a young woman who made this mistake and the terrible price both he and the young woman paid.

"I was very young and I was seeing a very nice young woman who was also quite sensitive. She'd cry when we made love and I could feel that she was deeply in love with me. She'd tell me she loved me and, like a lot of men, I'd tell her the same thing back. But the truth was that I didn't have strong feelings for her, I just liked the sex.

"I was seeing other women. One day she found out and had a fit. I went home feeling very self righteous. I told myself that we'd never agreed not to see other people. If she thought we had a monogamous relationship, that was her problem.

"She tried to kill herself. A serious attempt. She was in a coma for days. I had to spend time with her parents in the hospital and explain to the police and the hospital staff what happened. I was only 20 at the time. It scared the hell out of me. Her brother hit me in the face when she finally came out of the coma. Her father gave me a look that tore my heart out. Finally, her mother took me aside and told me stories about how sensitive her daughter was, how little things would make her cry and fill her with pain. She said she never wanted me around her daughter again. If I saw her again, she'd send someone after me to hurt me.

"I learned a lesson that day the hard way. Never tell someone you love them if you don't, even if it causes the relationship to end. It ends up hurting people very badly when you lie, <u>very</u> badly."

Lynn, one of the women at the coffee shop, shakes her head. "My daughter tells me that every boy she goes out with says he loves her. I tell her they just want to get in her pants."

The ladies at the coffee shop whoop it up and when things settle down, Crystal says, "That's something you learn with age, doc. But most people now can't tell love from like. They feel so unloved that any little attention gets blown way beyond what it means. Kids today must be the most unloved people around cause they can't keep their feelings straight. One date and they're in love. It's pretty sick out there."

Honest men have a difficult time saying they love someone. That's because the word "love" is a serious word and it means something that, once said, can't be taken back. In the careful world healthy men live in, keeping such feelings inside until they're very sure about the other person is a way of life. But you can tell when a man is falling in love with you by his behavior. He may not say the "L" word, but his actions tell you that he's falling for you.

Men in love are solicitous and concerned about your feelings. They want to impress you and they take extra care in how they look when they're around you. Men in love give presents and try and involve themselves in your life. Men in love make longer term commitments and agree to plan for activities well into the future. They may never quite get the courage to tell you they love you but their behavior ought to let you know that they're going from liking to loving you.

Women can guide men by helping them learn the words that describe feelings of affection, intimacy, and love. Liking someone better than sliced bread is obviously not the same as saying that you're in love. Teach your men the language of affection and it will make life a lot easier for you since you'll know where you stand in a relationship.

Rule 4: Dangerous Men Will Rob You Of Your Soul

You deserve respect from the man you're with. If he's abusive or demeaning, if he breaks promises or seems emotionally cold, if he drinks too much, you're with a man who will not love you. Don't delude yourself, ladies, it's not going to happen. This kind of man, and there are plenty of them, thrives on the love women give them which they never give back. It's a game to them because, underneath it all, they don't much like women. They like the idea of conning and lying and seeing how much they can get away with.

They can be attractive and very charming, and when they con you, they might do it with style and ease so that it doesn't feel as if you're being conned. But you are. Make no mistake about it, as this story from one of the ladies at the coffee shop describes.

"I was going out with this real smooth operator. A real charmer. He could charm the skin off a snake. It was fun to be with him. People would gravitate over whenever we were together. He just seemed to have such charm, it was like a magnet. Then one night he accused me of saying something snide about him. He called me names and he beat me to a pulp. I've been lucky before. It's never happened to me. I thought he was going to kill me.

"You would think that he'd take a hike, wouldn't you, but there he was back in my life being so charming and apologetic that I fell for it. He talked to me about his family and how abusive they were. He bought me gifts and he took me places. It was like being on a honeymoon. Then one night, he nearly killed me. I learn fast and I stopped seeing him, but I know women who let this sort of thing happen all the time.

"Men who abuse women are dangerous. Stay away from them, that's what I tell my friends. Charming men are sometimes monsters. Don't fall for their line or it might be the end of your life. And if you think healthy guys are too boring, take my word for it. I'd rather be bored a little than beaten to a pulp. Anytime."

I have an entire chapter on men who abuse women later in the book. If you have a pattern of going out and getting involved with abusive men, look to your past. Often women who have patterns of involvement with abusers are women who themselves have been physically, emotionally, or sexually abused as children. In a crazy sort of way, these women find abusive men comfortable men to be with. The abusive behavior and the honeymoon period after the abuse are a comfortable, but dangerous form of love to them because early on in their lives, they began to confuse abuse with love.

If you have a pattern of dating and falling in love with abusive men, there are two things you must do immediately. One, stop seeing the man as quickly as possible and two, get professional help to stop the abuse cycle. If you don't, sooner or later you stand a very good chance of getting badly hurt, and I mean very badly hurt. The main reason for going to emergency rooms in America for women under 30 is physical abuse by men. Believe it, ladies, it's no joking matter.

Rule 5: Young Love And Other Sorrows: You're Not A Teenager Anymore. Don't Expect Your Man To Be One, Either

Early love is the strongest love, but not necessarily the best love. When we fall in love for the first time, nothing ever matches it again in intensity or power. But, after all, it may be very young love, or it may be love at a time when we aren't fully formed as human beings. Don't confuse young love with mature love. Don't compare your feelings for someone at a more mature time in your life with the love you may have felt for someone when you were younger. It can't possibly be the same kind of love.

This romantic view of love is the downfall of too many middle-aged men and women who think that love at 45 or 55 should feel exactly the same way it felt at 15. If it doesn't, then they reject it altogether. If you don't believe me, ladies, then read the personals sometime and see what women write about the sort of love they're looking for. Here are three ads written by older women taken at random from the LA Times:

"Romantic walks on the beach, nights in Rome, a get away weekend in paradise. If you're a man who can give me this, call…"

"Quiet talks over dinner, candle lights and a fire. I seek a man who will fulfill my destiny."

"Stars bursting in the night, love and intimacy like you've never known. I'm yours for the asking."

I'm not kidding. These are middle aged women. A man reading these ads would absolutely keel over laughing. Everyone knows that relationships are not like this, even if the movies say they are and even if you had a teen-aged love that came close. This sort of fantasy is a killer of love from a man's point of view. It exists inside the fevered brain of someone who doesn't understand mature love or mature men.

But men do the same thing. You'd be amazed at how many men still compare their high school sweethearts to their current love interests. It's called "High School Beauty Queen Syndrome" and every time I get together for a class reunion and see my old friends, I get an ear full of it. Listen to one of my old Grand Forks, North Dakota Central High School buddies talk about it:

"See Belinda over there? I've had the deep hots for her since I was 15. I've been married three times now. It must be the class record. Every woman I've been married to has had to measure up to Belinda. We do the things I used to do with her on dates. We go to similar movies. I tell the same jokes I told her. If they don't laugh, adios!

"I can't get over her. She's inside of me. I dream about her. She's still the prettiest cheerleader in the world and I'm still the hockey jock. We were the golden couple. That's what the yearbook called us, the golden couple. I wanted to marry her so bad, but she had other plans. She went to school and met some rich guy, and that was that. She was the best thing a poor kid like me could ever have. And now that I can't have her, she's so deep in my heart, I can't get her out.

"Every woman I've ever been involved with has looked like her in some way. I saw a shrink about it after my last marriage failed. He said that I'd never get rid of her until I saw her and told her how I felt. So I did it last night. She cried when I told her. She cried and she walked away and said, 'Why didn't you tell me, Donny? I feel the same way and here we are in our fifties and it's too late.' Now she won't talk to me at all and I feel like warmed over death. I didn't think I was in her league anymore when she went to college. I figured I was some flunky guy who worked on the railroad and she wouldn't be interested in me. What a jerk I was. Now I'm more confused than ever. I don't know <u>what</u> to do."

I do. Start acting your age, Donny. Start living your life as if you were 55 instead of 15. And stop comparing all women to some inaccurate fantasy you have of a love that took place 40 years ago. And if you can't do it by yourself, get some help.

The ladies at the coffee shop all applaud my bravado, but they all have a wistful look on their face. Young love and other sorrows, who can ever forget?

Rule 6: Men Sometimes Look For Women Who Are Like Their Mothers

It may be a little corny to say so, but men often look for women who are, in important ways, just like their mothers. Often they use the ways mothers treated them as guides to what they're looking for in a woman to love. And just as often, women try and act like a man's mother, even if it isn't sincere.

My advice is to never get into an arrangement like this with a man. It can only lead to unhappiness. Look for the man who likes you for who you are, not for the man who needs you to be his mother. In healthy relationships, men and women often pattern some of the qualities they look for in a mate after their parents. But they are the good qualities, the qualities of trust, loyalty, and commitment. When you pattern relationships after the troubling aspects of parents, as these examples will suggest, then you may be in deep trouble.

I had a male client whose mother was ill throughout my client's childhood. She had three children who largely raised themselves without the mother's help. His father was an overworked fellow who hardly kept his head above water throughout those terrible years. What my client did when he became an adult was to fall in love with someone very frail who developed health problems. He did a much better job of caring for his children than his father, but the situation was essentially the same.

"I don't know that I did it consciously," he says, "but there was a side of me that wanted to recreate the life I lived as a kid and to put myself in my dad's place, but do a better job. Well, I did that. I took care of a sick wife and three children. I did a great job at it, too. And you know what? Like my dad, I resented my wife and kids. It took my life away and left me without good memories. I proved that I could do a better job than my dad, but I wasn't any happier than he was and maybe, in a way, I was a lot sadder. I'd say to any man or woman who tries to imitate the relationship their parents had, that imitation doesn't let you to have your own unique life. How can anyone be happy imitating someone else's life?

Another client of mine told me that his parents had the ideal love relationship. He remembers his mother as a dashing, beautiful woman who always dressed formally for dinner and his father as a handsome, athletic man who was always perfect in the way he looked and acted. It was a sort of Jay Gatsby existence, as my client recalls.

"I saw the movie The Great Gatsby and I knew that was the way it had to be in my life because that was the way it was when I was growing up in this rich home in Kansas City. The only problem was that I could never get anyone to play the role of Daisy the way my mother played it. Women called me a snob because of the way I wanted them to be and to dress. I figured I was doing this great, romantic thing.

"Finally, I met the perfect Daisy. She was the ideal model of my mother. She loved to dress up and to be the perfect hostess. I was in love beyond description. And then I began to recognize that my perfect love was an alcoholic, just, god help me, like my mother. Only I'd denied that my mother had a drinking problem. But being around my perfect woman brought it all back to me. I was in anguish. It couldn't possibly be O.K. to be married to a lush. It was too much of an embarrassment and a reminder of what my home life really was like. It's amazing how people remember what they want to remember. I couldn't ever think of my mother as having a problem. For me, she was the perfect woman, but she wasn't, of course. Not by a long shot."

Rule 7: He's Got The World On A String, And You're On The Other End

Don't lose your identity in a relationship by letting the relationship dictate what you do, how you feel, or who you are. Too many women permit themselves to become so wrapped up in the glory of love that they slowly begin to lose their identities. Men love this feeling of control. It allows them to believe that they hold the power in a relationship. Permit a man to make you dependent on him and, in time, he will. He'll also resent you for it. Dependent women are boring to most men, and falling for a man who needs to control you will often end with the man resenting you for your weakness. Consider this story from a former female colleague:

"I was lost after Jack died. I couldn't make myself a cup of coffee or go to the store to shop. I do these complex things at work, but here I am at 48 and I can't even pay the bills or make simple decisions. As I look over my life with Jack, I can see that I gave up parts of myself to him. Many things I'd done before we got married, I stopped doing, completely. It wasn't only things I gave up, it was also beliefs, values, and interests. I used to love movies, but since he didn't, I stopped seeing them. I can't even get myself to watch them now that he's gone. I used to ski, but he was afraid of getting hurt, so I don't ski anymore. I used to be a liberal, but he wasn't, so now I don't know where I stand on politics. I don't know what I'm supposed to believe, or think, or feel anymore. Now that he's gone, I can't seem to get in touch with anything. I feel like I'm floating through life. I talk to him at night hoping he'll tell me what to do but, of course, he's silent now. Maybe I can find someone like Jack again. He made my life so easy, it was effortless."

If a man equates love with control, it's time for you to either do some hard work to change his mind or to get yourself another man. Men like to think that making decisions for women is a masculine thing to do. It's not. The masculine thing to do is to let women develop in their own way without a man trying to subvert or direct their growth. That's a much more masculine thing to do than robbing women of their independence and dignity.

Rule 8: Gypsies, Tramps, And Thieves: Forget Em. Go For the Nice Guys

A lot of men have given up on women. These are the nice guys who have been hurt so often by the not so nice women out there that they want nothing to do with women anymore. Some of you may feel the same way about men, maybe with good reason. The tragedy is that loneliness is a killer. At some point in your life, when the kids are gone or when work stops occupying your time, men and women need relationships. Maybe friends can satisfy some of that need but, sooner or later, loneliness and the need for emotional intimacy begin to set in.

There's almost nothing worse in life than to reach that moment when you know that you'll never be intimate again with another person. Love, you tell yourself, will never happen. Listen to one of the men at the coffee shop talk about it:

"I was seeing this lady. She was lovely to me one minute and then she was a killer the next. She'd miss dates and not call me up in advance to tell me she wasn't coming. Days later she'd call up with some excuse, but I never trusted her at all. She told me she loved me right from the start. She'd wash my clothes but then she wouldn't show up for weeks and I'd have to buy new clothes. She wouldn't answer the phone or call me back if I left a message. One day she'd call and she'd have this horrible story about why she hadn't seen me, and she'd cry and plead for us to get together.

"I know you're thinking that I should have stopped seeing her the first time she acted crazy, but it isn't easy to give something up at my age. Loneliness is awful and the attention of a pretty woman made me feel happy for the first time in years. And when you've gone for a long time without sex, giving it up is pretty difficult. After six or seven of these nutty episodes, my gut felt like it would burst. I started thinking about going to her house and doing something really terrible to her. Finally, I screamed at her on the phone to leave me alone. I've never talked that way to anyone in my life. After about 20 calls pleading with me to get back with her, she finally gave up and she's left me alone. It makes me sick to think that I went out with someone so crazy. I haven't been able to go out with anyone since and it's been three years. I keep thinking that the next woman I go out with will be just as bad and I just couldn't take it again."

These men who have given up on women are the really nice guys you should befriend. If you can be nice and thoughtful, if you can recognize the hurt they've been through and treat them with sensitivity, you may have found someone really terrific to share your life.

Like them, don't give up. There really <u>are</u> good men out there if you're willing to spend some time looking and if you can understand that they match your hurt feelings about relationships, experience by experience. Treat them the way you want to be treated after being badly hurt and you may have just found yourself a lifelong soul mate.

Rule 9: Men, What Are They Good For?

Don't expect too much from men. Often men aren't romantic, loving, tender or particularly sexual. The moment pretty much determines how they will be. If they're upset or tired, they'll act that way. Men are not very good at hiding feelings. Not, ladies, nearly as good as you are. Women are taught to hide feelings. Men are taught to ignore feelings. Big difference.

Women are much better than men at being loving and tender, even when they don't feel like it. So the better way to deal with men is to set the rules from the beginning. If you want a loving and romantic partner, mister, then let's see the same thing from you. Expect more because you deserve it, but don't get upset if it doesn't happen right away. Men need to be educated. That ought to be your goal in a relationship. To teach them to be more caring, even when they don't feel that way.

One of the wise ladies at the coffee shop raises her hand (isn't it interesting that we still do this as adults?) and asks if she can tell a story. This is what she says: "My Ted was like a spoiled mama's boy when we got married. His mama did everything for him. The more she did the more he expected her to do. Same with me. I was his slave and he could treat me as bad as he wanted to. Those were his rules.

We had a bad first year of marriage. I almost walked out. I wasn't his slave. I wasn't his mama, either. I was his wife and I deserved respect. I wouldn't back down. We had some awful fights and then we did some good talking. We set up the rules for the way we were gonna be to each other. If we strayed from the rules, we could talk about it, and we did, a lot. After about a year, we could feel things getting real good between us. The fighting stopped and we would sit at home feeling this loving thing just come over us. He treats me like a queen now and I treat him like a king. We got no reason to fight anymore. It's worth fighting in the beginning when you know how good it's gonna be in the end."

Rule 10: The Rules Everybody Should Know About Men But Sometimes Don't

These are some additional things you should know already about dealing with men in the initial period of dating. I won't go into detail because they should be pretty self-evident. So here goes.

1) Don't be compulsively late for dates. It drives men absolutely crazy. They see it as insulting and inconsiderate. Don't do it to him and don't let him do it to you.

2) Don't talk compulsively on dates, even if you're nervous, and don't interrupt when your date is talking. Men find compulsive talking nerve racking. Keep the flow of the conversation going. If you really want to impress a man, ask questions which will let him talk about himself. Men love to brag about their achievements, but have very little opportunity to do it with other men.

3) If a man is supposed to call you at a certain time and day, be at home. If a man calls continually and you're not there, he'll assume you're with another man or that you don't really care about him, and he'll give up. If you've been out late for reasons other than a date, call back as soon as possible and give him the reason you were out. It may seem unnecessary to you, but if you aren't at home and if you don't call back as soon as possible, you can expect him to give up on you.

4) Be honest about other men in your life. If they're just friends, explain this to a man you're dating. If you're involved with someone but it's cooling off and about to end, be up front with a man or he'll be very hurt because you haven't been honest with him. And expect the man to be equally honest with you.

5) This is the day and age of sexually transmitted diseases and AIDS. Be safe in your sexual practices. Don't let an older man have unprotected sex with you just because you think older men are safer. In many ways, older men are more dangerous because they've had more partners over the years. Ask for their sexual histories before having sex and be safer by using condoms. Many people feel, and I agree, that before having sex, you should both be tested for the HIV Positive Virus and other sexually transmitted diseases as a precaution.

6) Don't get involved with married men. It's dumb and it'll hurt in the long run. It's also ethically wrong. Just as you would be hurt if your husband were involved with someone else, someone's wife is going to get hurt. In the long run, all you have to measure your life by is how ethical you've been with others. Having an affair with a married man is a decidedly not nice thing to do. If God is watching, and he is, you can bet that it'll count against you.

7) Don't lead men on and don't lie about your feelings. If a man thinks you feel strongly about him, but you don't, it will hurt him very badly. See rule number 6 for how it will set with God.

8) Don't set your standards so high that it will be impossible to find a man who will match them. Life is short. Before you know it, the pool of men will have dwindled considerably. Set realistic standards for who you date, and don't turn

off the large number of men who may be very good for you, but don't absolutely look, feel, and act like your ideal man.

9) Don't come on like gangbusters and give men gifts too early in the relationship. It will just serve to make them gun shy. Give gifts that are appropriate when they should appropriately be given. Birthdays and Father's Day are good examples. Don't start throwing money at a man you barely know. It will only scare him off or set up unrealistic expectations for the future.

10) Don't make a man feel embarrassed by putting him down over insignificant things. I knew a woman who said, after she'd had dinner with a friend of mine and the check was on the table, that she measured a man's desirability by how much he left for a tip. The tip my friend gave her after they left the restaurant was, "Adios and good riddance."

And The Ladies Have The Last Word

The ladies at the coffee shop nod or shake their heads as I finish my short lecture. We sit for awhile thinking about the rules of engagement and then I look at my watch and tell everyone it's time to leave. I have to teach an early morning class.

As I walk away, somebody at the table says that what I've told them is worth thinking about. As I'm almost out the door and out of sight, I can hear one of them say, "I still think men are screwy. And men in love are the worst." What can I say? Men are screwy when they're in love. But if you understand them and if you make an effort to walk life in a man's shoes, you'll find the experience very rewarding. Love is everything it's cracked up to be. Approach it with wisdom and it will never cease to amaze you.

6

Why the Caged Bird Doesn't Sing Anymore: Men and Their Marriage Blues

Lonely When Single, Miserable When Married

Everyone of the women I meet at the coffee shop is, or has been married. While they may complain bitterly about their men, all of them admit that marriage beats being single, although a few of them aren't entirely sure. As Leona, the lone Black participant in our discussions says, "I'm still feeling too giddy being out of my marriage to say that it's better than being single. Right now, it's a relief, but maybe in awhile it'll get lonely. I like the institution of marriage even if the men are sometimes pretty lame."

Jackie, a semi-regular nods her head. "It's good to be with another person at my age. Sometimes it's boring, you know, but then, so is being by yourself. I'd take being married any day over being single again. And you've got family around you, and that can be a comfort."

And so the debate goes. Most people in America <u>do</u> get married. But then, a significant number of them get divorced. Not once or twice, but three times or more. We seem to be pretty confused about marriage as a condition of adult life.

To add to our confusion, we can't seem to stay faithful once we're married. 70% of the married men and 30% of the married women of America are unfaithful to their spouses. And that's a conservative estimate, particularly for the married women. It comes from the Kinsey report in the 1950's. Most people think the infidelity rate is much higher now.

For many of us, marriage is a sweet experience full of good moments. For those lucky men who have good marriages, nothing is ever better in their lives. Children usually result from marriages. The experience of raising a child in a loving home with two adults who have a mature and trusting relationship is one of the most thrilling and powerful experiences any man can have in his life.

Most men have had moments in their married life that are idyllic. Good times in marriage are strong reasons to stay married in bad times and to re-marry as an alterative to being single.

Married life, when it's good, compliments the best parts of us. We feel better being with another person than we feel alone. Important issues in our lives can be discussed with a caring spouse, and the decisions we make are often better than if we'd made them on our own.

Because of all of this, married people are generally physically and emotionally healthier. For all of the negative things we say about marriage, married people do better than single people, particularly better than older single men who often flounder and fail in their lives because loneliness takes its toll on a man's physical and emotional health. Men have the highest rates of suicide in America and men over 65 commit suicide at ever increasing rates.

And yet, the data are clear. Marriages don't work well in America. If they did, then the coming together of two, and three, and sometimes four families as a result of a new marriage wouldn't take place. We wouldn't have the domestic violence problems we have in America. The infidelity and divorce rates wouldn't be as high as they are. And certainly, the men of America would be at home helping to raise their children instead of having abandoned families so that single mothers and their children often live in a condition Mimi Abramowitz calls, "The feminization of poverty."

Why are marriages in so much trouble in America? And, more to the point, what can we do to strengthen and support marriage so that the results of marriages gone bad aren't so devastating to the men, women, and children of America, and <u>particularly</u> the children of America?

<u>I. Marriage is a Crap Shoot</u>

Anna, one of the regulars at the coffee shop is dating a new man, but she's hesitant about where the relationship is going. "I don't know," she says, "he's a nice guy and all, but we've both been burned in the past. I feel like we're holding back, you know? Neither of us wants to make a commitment to the other. We avoid the subject of going out with other people even though I don't think either of us is. I don't know. You mention commitment and marriage to a man and you're in trouble."

Crystal, the attractive lady who winks at me from time to time says, "Listen, honey, been there, done that. Marriage beats the hell out of running around in bars and meeting up with scum you wouldn't want to let use your bathroom at home. If I had a good man in my life," and she looks over at me and watches the little twitch in my eye, "I'd treat him so good that he'd never look at another woman so long as he lives. And that, ladies, is a fact."

Everyone nods. Marriage, it seems, beats the pants off the alternatives. But why, someone asks, do good people hurt each other so much in marriage? Why do so many good people run into trouble?

Marjorie, the waitress who hovers over us comes over to fill my cup with hot coffee and to leave a large hot sticky bun with butter in front of me. Bribes. We all watch the butter run down the sticky bun and onto the plate. It's a beautiful sight so early in the morning.

This is what I tell them as I munch on my hot sticky bun which, by the way, is delicious beyond description and will wreck my new diet.

II. Young Marriage Decisions Are Often Bad

Most of us marry when we're young. Our interests and needs are not fixed. We often go into marriages without having mature sensibilities and, as a consequence, we make bad mistakes. Evidence exists that the older a man or a woman are when they marry, the more likely the marriage will be successful and last. This suggests that maturity of partners is a very important ingredient in a successful marriage.

My friend Jim Schefter, who has since passed away, wrote a great book on the Corvette and used to argue with me that people follow patterns in their relationships that can't be overcome. Unconscious issues determine who we are attracted to and our choices in mates. If we've done badly at 20, some psychological imperative will drive us to do badly at 50. And yet, even though he believed that, he also thought that the true and real love of his life would take him into old age. I believe that time is a great leveler of immaturity. As we get older, we learn from the past and we gain wisdom in our choices of mates. Hopefully!

III. The Crunching Boredom of Marriage

Many of us get bored in marriage, even with the right person, chosen at the right time, and for all the right reasons. The day to day toll of being with someone can be tremendous. Who among us has not felt a surge of guilt when we find ourselves idly thinking about other people, even though our spouses are as wonderful as they can be? It's certainly the way men think. Some men control their passions and stay happily with one women, while others stray like ally cats on the prowl. No one is proud of it. No one wishes it on their worst enemy. But it happens, and it happens a lot.

Men always need to prove themselves. One way they do this is by looking for women to reaffirm that they are still attractive, intelligent, and sexually potent. Men don't stray to search for love and intimacy, they stray because they have a need to continually prove themselves. When a man describes an affair and says that it meant nothing, that he didn't love the person he slept with, he's not lying. The person probably <u>didn't</u> mean anything other than to confirm his need for a conquest. Now he can beat his chest, give out an old Tarzan war cry, and feel like he's king of the jungle for a day or two.

Nice behavior? Of course it isn't. It demeans women and it's hurtful. In this life, betrayal is one of the worst things that anyone can do to a loved one. Men destroy relationships because they're insecure about themselves. Having affairs is not something secure men do, it's a thing immature and insecure men do to answer an unanswerable question they repeatedly pose: "Will this attractive woman be smitten with me? And so smitten, will she honor me with a roll in the hay?" It's like preparing for battle in a way. It isn't about love or affection, it's about the conquest of another human being.

IV. The Business Of Marriage Is Business

Marriage can become very complicated. Having children, buying and selling homes and cars, financial pressures, all of it can be very stressful. Many married couples over-extend ourselves when times are good only to find that they can't make it financially when times are bad. Children may have special needs that occupy a couple's time and are taxing financially. Illness may be an unfortunate occurrence which can change our lives. Love can be severely challenged when stress levels in marriage are high. Listen to what my ex-client Jeff had to say about his marriage.

"I'm not happy to admit it, but after so many years of doing business together, of buying and selling stuff, my wife felt more like a business partner than a lover. It's difficult to think of a business partner as someone to cuddle up with in bed. We'd go for long periods of time without sex. Neither of us minded, I don't think, because we no longer felt any passion. "It just seems to me that so many of us in modern marriages let the passion slip away because we get caught up in buying and selling things. Junk, really, stuff to occupy ourselves so that we don't have to look at how lousy our marriages have become. As far as I'm concerned, once marriage feels like a business thing, you can kiss it off. It's dead."

The ladies at breakfast nod their heads when they hear this story. Ginny, a dispatcher for a truck company who is usually very quiet, looks up and says, "That sure sounds like me and the old man. We buy and sell stuff and we're busy all the time with the kids. But there are times when I feel like I'm still at work for all the love and romance in our marriage."

Everyone looks down at their coffee. It's unanimous. Marriage can suck the tenderness right out of you if you let it.

V. I'm Stressed Out And I Feel As Sexy As A Prune

We may feel so overwhelmed by the pressures in our lives that we become thoughtless and inconsiderate to our mates. Modern life is demanding. Being able to maintain a relationship when we're under pressure at work or in our private lives can be difficult, even for those couples who are deeply in love, as this story from a former client will confirm.

"I was working this out of town job. I had to do a lot of flying around the country and it was really draining. I'd come home from a trip and my wife would be happy to see me. She'd fix a special meal or make everything really romantic. But I wasn't in the mood. I was dog tired from the trips and irritable as hell at her for making demands on me to be nice. All I wanted to do was to sit down, have a drink, and look at television. I was never very good at telling her this and I used to try and act nice to her, but it didn't take long for her to see that my heart wasn't in whatever she had planned. After a year or two, she stopped trying.

"When someone you're married to stops trying, it's the kiss of death. Everything just stopped working for us. I wish I'd chucked the damn job. I lost a very good woman, the best I'll ever have in my life. You could say that it was because of the job, but I didn't do anything to change the situation. I could have, but I wanted to feel like a martyr, the hard working husband whose wife puts too much pressure on him. Stress is a killer, alright, but how you handle it can make or break a relationship. I realize now that I should have gotten help, but I was young, cocky, and thoughtless. See where it got me?"

VI. Renewal Isn't Only For Library Cards

Most of us don't have ways to periodically improve our relationships. Like everything in life, relationships need to be worked on if they're to succeed. Many couples incorrectly believe that the work on a marriage needs to be done during courtship. But to really make a marriage work, couples must constantly fix the small and large problems that plague a marriage, and they have to learn to recapture a loving and committed concern for one another. A friend of mine put it this way:

"Somewhere along the line, we lost it. I don't know how and I'm not sure when it happened, but gradually we lost our love and it hasn't come back. Neither of us knows what to do about it. We sit and argue about money when we can't talk about the fact that we haven't slept together in months. We fight about the kids when we can't discuss the fact that our bodies no longer arouse us. We scream at each other about little problems that should annoy us, not drive us into a rage.

"We give impersonal birthday presents to one another: lawn mowers, steak knives, tools, presents that offend and hurt our feelings. And finally, like old couples who sleep in separate rooms, we call each other "father" and "mother" in some awful reversal of roles that confuses our children who aren't sure now what to call us anymore. You've got to work on a relationship all the time or it can become pretty boring and routine. You can't feel special about someone when your lives together are routine and boring."

VII. Affairs Kill Any Chance For Love

The risk of meeting someone else who seems better able to meet our needs is very great when marriages are in trouble. Other people often become attractive to us, particularly when our feelings for our spouses are at their lowest point. These excursions into other relationships can be very damaging, even if we never act physically on them. Infidelity takes a toll on the very notions of love and commitment, notions that form the basis of marriage. Many men believe that they can have affairs and maintain relationships in marriage. It's nonsense. Most wives know and are hurt and angered by infidelity, just as men are devastated by a wife's infidelity. There is a wonderful moment in the film, <u>Wolf</u> when Jack Nicholson begins developing the senses of a wolf and smells a colleague's scent on his wife's coat. In that moment he knows of his wife's infidelity and, like a wounded animal, he bounds across town to confront the couple. Every man who dreams of being unfaithful should see that scene and remember that when we've been in a marriage for a long time, our husbands and wives develop a sixth sense about us that can catch us in all sorts of lies, deceits, and untruths.

When Marriages Are in Trouble

No one who's gone through a marital problem wants to do it again. The level of anger and the feelings of betrayal many of us experience can make life miserable. When marriages are in difficulty, men and women say things to each other that may lead to years of arguments and hard feelings even after the couple separates or divorces. And remember, there is no such thing as a true divorce from marriage if you have children, property, and mutual friends. Couples who hate each other may have to continue speaking for years to work out arrangements for visitations, college, and a variety of issues that concern us as parents.

While you may feel that there is nothing to resolve when a marriage is failing, there is a great deal of evidence that marital therapy with a competent therapist can save marriages. There is further evidence that marital therapy and divorce mediation can help divorcing couples get along better after the divorce.

In several studies of divorce mediation, divorce agreements were maintained at a 90% rate when mediation was used as opposed to 25% of the time when adversarial proceedings using opposing lawyers were used. The only ones who come out of a contested divorce better off are the opposing lawyers. Divorce agreements are frequently broken in contested divorces and couples are forced back into court to resolve minor problems that the court can legally resolve but can't, or won't, enforce.

"So what do you do when your marriage starts to go sour?" one of the women at the coffee shop asks after a brief discussion of how things can go very wrong, even in the best of marriages. We fill our cups with coffee. I look at my watch. It's 6:15 AM and the sun is beginning to come up over the large arrow on the mountain facing the coffee shop which gives Lake Arrowhead its name. For a moment, we look at the sight. It dazzles everybody and, for the hundredth time or so, I remember why we all live in California even when crime and smog and a thousand other problems can make life miserable.

I look around at the ladies and I'm surprised to see a few of the nearby men pull up their chairs and join us. Further down the row of tables is a small prayer meeting. I can see the bowed heads of four men in prayer and silently wish them well. This is what I suggest.

Don't Let The Ship Sink Without a Struggle

I. Confronting Trouble

Be sensitive to the changes in a relationship and try to confront your man about them. Be specific. Don't talk about love or sensitivity. Mention spending less time together or how too much of your free time is spent on issues other than the relationship. Be very specific when giving feedback about the behavior that concerns you. Men are best when you give them direct information. And don't be "brow beaten" out of your perception of a problem. Stick to your guns and consider the way a former client handled a confrontation with her husband when their relationship began to drift.

"It wasn't anything really specific that I was noticing, you know, we just seemed to be drifting away from each other. We weren't talking much anymore. We were together, but we really weren't. So I just pointed it out to him. I said that we seemed to be drifting apart. I gave him examples of how we'd stopped talking very much. At first he disagreed, but the more I wouldn't let it slide, the more he listened. We started to talk and, to my surprise, there were also major problems from his point of view. It wasn't just little things, either. He wasn't sure he loved me anymore.

"We went for help to a marriage counselor and that cleared the air some, but it still wasn't quite right between us. It took two years of constant hard work and talking to sort it out, but we did it. I think we didn't know each other very well before we got married. Neither one of us had the ability to deal with conflict. I'm glad I stuck with it, though. I love my husband and I think he loves me. We're in much better shape now. If we hadn't started to talk about problems in our relationship, we'd be just another divorced American couple. That simple."

II. Men Resent Being Treated Like Children

Many of the women I work with consider their spouses to be spoiled brats, little babies, one-dimensional beings with hardly an idea in their heads about the reasons a marriages isn't working. But they're surprised to discover how aware men can be in therapy or in court. When payback time comes, you may be appalled at how mean your man can be for the years of being treated so badly, as this story from a colleague of mine demonstrates.

"You know Judy. A more opinionated woman never walked the face of the earth. There was nothing she didn't know and no one she wouldn't tell it to. In time, that woman turned me into dog shit. She just kept brow beating me until I stopped having an opinion about anything. I just gave up on the marriage. She could have her way every time. It wasn't worth hearing that whinny voice of hers argue with me. God, I really hated her.

"When I'd had enough, I got the meanest divorce lawyer who ever walked the face of the earth. I went for custody of the kids and as much of her savings as I could get. In court, I wasn't the meek little academic she'd grown to believe that I was. No, sir. My lawyer worked with me for weeks to make me assertive and tough. And I was. Really tough. And mean. And dirty. I said things in court that were such lies I thought that my nose would fall off. And you know something? The more I lied, the better I felt. When it was over, we destroyed her. Ripped her heart out. I was so overcome with emotions, I kissed my lawyer. Judy just sat looking at me when it was over. She didn't think I had the balls to do it. It was one of the happiest moments of my life to see her that way."

If you treat men like children, if your opinion of your husband is so bad that you think he's incapable of change, don't be surprised if a moment comes when he's had enough and he does something extreme. If you can't work with him to change, if you've given up on him, that's the time to be thinking about divorce. But if you're angry and want the little bugger to suffer some, remember about payback time. There are a number of people who believe that abandonment of children and unwillingness of men to honor child support agreements are all about payback for bad treatment in the marriage. You may disagree, I certainly do, but many men feel that way, nonetheless.

III. A Marital Therapist Is Cheaper Than A Lawyer, And A Lot Nicer

Hiring a good therapist to help work out problems in the relationship saves a lot of money and stress down the pike. While they may not help save the marriage, they may help resolve the anger and hurt that accompany marital problems, and they may help make the divorce saner. Not all therapists are created equal; some are really very poor. Ask around for the names of good people and respect the information of friends who have gone through marital therapy. Check with your medical plan for the coverage you have since medical insurance and employee assistance plans at work may pay for most of the cost. Above all, listen to what a friend of mine had to say about going for therapy:

"I've got to tell you right up front, Glicken, that I think therapy is for the birds. One of the truly silly inventions in a truly silly age. I have this image of talking to some overweight woman who has tissues all over the place in case you cry. In my family, we worked it out on our own. That's the way it was with my marriage. I was working it out on my own, but I was really bungling it. The more I worked, the worse things got. And I was drinking too much. It was pretty messy time in my life.

"I went to my doctor for a check up because I wasn't feeling well. My blood pressure was off the scale. My cholesterol was higher than ever. I was a wreck. He made me go, kicking and screaming I might add, to a therapist. He said if I didn't go, that he'd recommend withdrawing my medical insurance for lack of compliance with his medical advice. I knew he was bluffing, but it was all that it took to get me to go.

"And I hated it. The therapist was a creep. The sessions were so rummy that I'd laugh about it all the way home. The guy was really dumb, I thought, until one day he got mad at me for being such a smart ass and he nailed me. He told me what I was doing, why I was doing it, where it was going to lead me, and to get the hell out of his office and not to come back until I was serious about changing since there were people out there with real problems, not smart alecky academics like me who were such wise guys they thought they knew everything when, in fact, they knew squat.

"He really kicked me out. I went home a little shaken. No one had talked to me that way since I was a kid. I sat at home thinking about what he'd said. He was absolutely right about everything. I called him up the next day and apologized, and asked if I could come back. He agreed but said that there had to be some pain involved or I'd dog it the way I had before. He made me pay the full fee, $150 an hour and no insurance co-pay. He said he'd think about a refund, but only if I worked hard. He said he was going to kick my ass from here to China since it seemed to be all I could understand. And he did. I mean he said some things to me that made me come close to punching him out. But you know what? They were all true and they needed to be said. I pulled in my pride and I listened. And it helped. It helped so much I can never repay him for the way my life changed.

"Gina and I have a wonderful thing now. It's better than I should ever have, given the stuff we found out about the way I relate to women, the really shitty attitude I have about them. Going to a therapist saved my life. I don't know about other men, but it turned me around real fast. Maybe a lot of men feel the same way about therapy that I did. I don't know what to say to them except to find someone who will be honest with you and work very hard. It can make a really big difference in your life."

IV. Divorce Mediation

If you've come to the point where it's clear that your marriage is going to fail, and heaven help us, that's a realization that can be all but inevitable in some marriages, don't hire an attorney at first. Seek out a divorce mediator. Most mediators are trained therapists with special training in negotiating divorce settlements.

Attorneys can write the agreement in legal language and file the agreement with the appropriate court, but the divorce agreement itself may become impossible when attorneys get you to argue over issues. The only people who benefit from disagreements in divorces are attorneys. Whether you like it or not, suck in your pride, find a mediator, and work out a fair agreement. You'll have to deal with your spouse, if you have children, for the rest of your life. Better think about that when you're going for the other person's juggler, and think about this story from a male client who, thankfully, sought help from a mediator instead of slogging it out in court.

"I knew this divorce would kill me financially. I also knew that I couldn't win anything. In the state I lived in, the woman gets everything, even if she's the sister of Satan. So I suggested that we see a mediator. I offered to pay the bill. For the kid's sake and to keep us on reasonable terms, my wife agreed. It was a great experience. We worked everything out by compromising. Neither of us came out of it feeling cheated. I found myself being much more generous. To my surprise, my wife turned out to a lot less mean. She could have killed me financially.

"As it turned out, in about ten hours, we negotiated all of the points of the divorce, signed an agreement, and took the agreement to an attorney to put in legal language. The mediator cost $1,000 and the lawyer charged $500 to write up the divorce papers and file them for us. The divorce would have cost $15,000-$25,000 for each of us if we'd used lawyers. We wouldn't have been better off and our relationship, after the divorce, would have been a mess. I figured that whatever the divorce would have cost if we'd used lawyers, we could put that money into the children. So I factored that savings into the child support agreement and increased the amount of child support. Better my kids get the money than an attorney, any day."

V. Staying Together For The Children

Is there anything wrong with staying in a marriage for the sake of the children? Only you can answer that question but, from my point of view, the answer is no, there isn't anything wrong, provided that you have respect for one another, treat each other well, and that your personal differences don't affect the children. Divorce isn't fun for anyone. The people we often date after a divorce are frequently not nearly as good as our spouses, and children do better in intact homes. From every study I've ever read, most of us are happier being married than divorced, as a former client reports who decided to stay with his wife for the sake of the children.

"We did all the stuff you're supposed to do. We went to an attorney and a therapist. We went on marriage retreats. We had long talks and wrote divorce decrees, but we just didn't have feelings for one another anymore. But when push came to shove, we couldn't see breaking up the family. We talked about having an open marriage where we could see other people, but neither of us had the heart to do it.

"We settled into a nice routine. I saw my friends, spent good time with my kids, took up some great hobbies that I'm still into and, guess what? We started to realize that we were still in love. It was a shock. I felt like I was being unfaithful at first. Here I was having an affair with my wife and I felt giddy and wonderful. We were supposed to be celibate, that was the agreement, but we were having this great physical relationship, so much better than we'd ever had before. It was sort of mind boggling.

"Our kids are happy and doing well, which is more than I can say for the children of other divorced couples we know. We're doing really well, now, too. We're a mature couple and it feels right to come home at the end of the day to my wife. I hope other men don't go off half cocked and leave their families. It's the worst feeling in the world to leave children and to throw away your life. If it were me telling other men what to do, I'd tell them to stay with it. Get help, do a lot of talking, but stay together. It sure beats being out there beating the bushes for relationships my single friends tell me are next to impossible to find."

VI. Staying With Marriage For The Long Haul

Marriage is a commitment. One way to keep it from moving toward divorce is to decide, in advance, that it will work. Research on couples who have been married 50 or more years conducted at Long Island University by Florence and Clyde Matthews (Modern Maturity, May-June 1995, p.92) suggests that couples who stay together for very long periods of time have a deep commitment to one another and very positive moral and societal values. Interestingly enough, many of the couples studied had persevered through multiple troubles including bankruptcy, alcoholism, infidelity, and chronic illness to then regain a sense of happiness and satisfaction with one another.

Equally interesting are the following findings: men described their marriages more positively than women. 60% of men versus 51.5 % of the women said that they were very happy in their marriages. 73% of the men versus 50% of the women said they always liked one another. Either women are the workers in longer marriages, or it is the man's positive view of his spouse and their marriage that generates long-term commitment.

An older man I know who's been married in excess of fifty years told me that the secret to a long marriage was to consider, in his words, that it was, "A done deal." By that he meant that once you marry, you did it for life. If you keep telling yourself that, you'll stay married through the worst of times.

"I wasn't the greatest husband all those years," he reports. "I strayed, had my flings, and I gambled from time to time and lost money. My wife resented the hell out of it, too. She wasn't so easy to live with all of the time. We had our share of problems and we didn't always handle them well, but something in us just wouldn't let the marriage end. We had kids and we had property and friends. We didn't want to lose our life, I guess.

"And then an amazing thing happened. We fell in love all over again after the kids left home. We rediscovered each other and it made our commitment even stronger. I don't see this happening much anymore. Young people have no commitment. If it isn't working out, they just leave. If you want to make a marriage last, you make a promise to yourself that you'll work at it and, with luck, you make it. We did. Here I am an old codger and I have a happier marriage than most young people. It sure is a good way to approach old age."

VII. Marriage May Not Be Perfect But It Beats The Heck Out of The Alternatives

Marriage may not be "rock n' roll," as they say out on the ski slopes, but it beats the heck out of anything else, particularly as we get older. Married friends often talk about the freedom of being single as if it were the most wonderful thing to ever happen in the history of the world. But it isn't always so great to be absolutely free to do whatever you want to do because, much of the time, you do it by yourself. Friends don't know how gut churning it is to think that you've found someone good and true only to discover that they have serious problems, or what it's like to make huge decisions without anyone else's help. I'm afraid they also fail to recognize that people often treat divorced folks like lepers, and divorced single folks like flesh eating lepers. As my divorced friend Jim once told me:

"The only people who like being single in middle age are the people who haven't a clue about what it's really like. They're the people right out of a marriage who think it's going to be easy. It takes them a year or so to get the picture, and then they settle into the routine of single life: the meals eaten alone, the nights of not being able to sleep so you start to talk to yourself, the awful people who call when you're asleep because they think a 1:00 AM call is romantic, the money thrown away on meaningless dates. If I could do it over again, I'd be better at marriage.

"I never thought being single again would be like this. I thought it would be cool, and exciting, and dramatic. It's not. It's lonely, and it's boring, and it's tough for a man my age to be alone so much of the time. No one who goes through a divorce ever wants to do it again, I can tell you that for certain."

VIII. It's Not Over Until It's Over

When it's over emotionally and you both know it, have the grace and wisdom to let go. Staying in a marriage when you're both doing harm to one another is just not wise. The fights, the bad feelings, the recrimination, all of it destroys the potential to have a healthy relationship in the future. When you've reached the point where you both know that the time is right to end the relationship, then you should do it, just as a friend reports in the following story:

"We've been separated for months now. She lives in one of our rental homes and I live in our house. It's a comfortable arrangement in many ways. I see her maybe 70% of the week, but it's making me wonder if I'm married or not. I feel like I'm in limbo. If we plan something, I never know until the last minute if she'll do it. She wants her space. I thought I was giving her space. When a woman talks about needing space, you know she's thinking divorce.

"I went on a trip recently with a lady friend, a wonderful person I've known for a long time. It made me realize that I want to get on with my life and that I hate this feeling I have of floating in space. Martha and I talked last night and decided that we ought to end things and get on with our lives. We cried a lot, too. And the awful thing is that I still love her, even though I know it isn't going to work. If she changed her mind and wanted us to try again, I'd be happy. She's a wonderful woman, but she won't change her mind. It's over, but a little of me keeps thinking that it might work again. I'm sure that'll change in time, but right now, I feel pretty awful. It's never a good feeling to think the person you loved, that maybe you <u>still</u> love, doesn't love you anymore."

And The Ladies Have The Last Word

The men and women gathered around the table look down at their feet. They've all been there before. It's old territory to them, but it hurts to think of a marriage gone bad. We finish our coffee in silence and, one by one, we stroll off to meet another California day. The sun is bright over the San Bernardino Mountains and the desert wind has blown the air crystal clear. Off by her truck, Crystal looks over at me and smiles a glorious smile, and it dawns on me for the thousandth time or so that this man/woman thing is the greatest. If we could make it work better, wouldn't that be incredible, wouldn't that be about the best thing any of us ever accomplished in our lives? That, as they used to say at my house when I was growing up, would be something to write home about.

Crystal waives at me as I get into my old Chevy and yells across the parking lot, "Have a great day, doc. You deserve one." Then she drives off in her pick up truck, a legacy from one of her marriages, head held high and posture ram rod straight. I watch her drive away and think to myself, what a wonder it is to have come through the hard times Crystal has had in her life and to still be a decent, kind, and loving person. It's a mystery to me since the same experiences would make most of us bitter and cruel.

We come to a stop light, side by side, and she rolls down the window. "It's time you got yourself a real woman, doc. Someone who will keep the house clean and take care of you at night. Think about it. Your book would write itself with a good woman there for you."

The light changes and we drive our separate ways. Well, of course. Why hadn't I thought of that?

7

Have Gun, Will Travel: Lies Men Tell Themselves to Cope with Divorce

Summertime Children

In the summer, the divorced men of America shuttle their children back and forth across the country for the annual ritual of summer vacation with their children. If you are in your middle years and your children are in a growth spurt, it feels as if the changes are too much to handle. One minute a child looks like a child, the next minute they're young men or women asking to drive the car.

For the lonely single men in America, summers with their children is like a moment of glory. For a month or two, life is sweet again. Someone laughs at your bad jokes and listens to your fears, your hopes, your dreams. This annual ritual of summer vacations is not without its painful side. You get accustomed to having someone else in the house, but when vacation is over, the loneliness you feel can be heartbreaking.

Many of the divorced men in America feel as if life is over for them. They know that they will never experience family life again or the sweet and tender moments of love. Their experiences as single men confirm a growing belief that the single women in the core group they date will only complicate their lives. This realization is a profound sorrow for most of them.

Much too late, many men wish they'd been better husbands and fathers. If they knew at 30 what they know at 50, they would have worked very hard to keep their families together. But many men, particularly men in their middle years, fear commitment and relationships because the pain of divorce and the dislocation of loved ones make them shy away from love and tenderness, just as they claim it is the very thing they want.

This fatalistic view of relationships is a deathblow to love and romance. It destroys that intangible and illusive experience. One needs an illusion, a dream, to allow love to happen, but an increasing number of single men in their middle years, their peak years, feel a lessening of hope. There is little to look forward to so why bother at all?

When these men re-marry or find someone to share the good moments of life, they often hold back emotionally, causing their wives and lovers to inundate the counselors and therapist of America to help them understand how best to deal with their husbands or boyfriends. It's a difficult task dealing with men who can't love or trust. Second and third marriages often end in divorce, as a result. Those of us who are interested in the lives of men know how deathly afraid men are to self-disclose, how they almost never seek help when they're in turmoil. We know that they turn to alcohol and drugs and, when all else fails, suicide to resolve hurts so deep and painful that even a good therapist can only scratch the surface.

The wives and lovers of these emotionally frozen men paint dismal pictures of their men, whom they view, finally, as children. They speak in terms of "little man" and "child" and "baby" when they discuss their husbands or lovers. As one listens to them it becomes clear how many men are physically present in a relationship, but increasingly their inner thoughts are deeply private. They seem alone, preoccupied, lost in a private dialogue that makes them seem inaccessible.

And so, with summer, these men reach inside for the love, the intense pride they feel for their children. If they are very, very lucky and if their children care deeply about them, it is a summer of discovery and joy. But if the private pain, the uncompromising and rigid nature of their thoughts keep them distant and aloof, the summer is one more indication to their estranged children of the unloving and uncaring nature of their fathers.

We live in hope and we hope for the best, but from where I sit in the isolated and detached atmosphere of Southern California, where fathers see children who live a mile or two away once or twice a year, or not at all, it looks as if many fathers have abdicated their roles and abandoned their children. I hope not. Many men work hard to keep the lines of love open with their children. Perhaps it is just the single men I see in restaurants with children, vacant-eyed and silent, who make me feel so pessimistic and sad.

Not Repeating Mistakes After Divorce

We're sitting in the coffee shop one rainy California morning. The gloom from the overcast and fog shroud the mountain and everyone looks sad and morose.

Weather is a constant in California, but when the sun leaves for a few days, everyone starts to feel adrift and anchorless.

Stephanie, one of the semi-regular members of the group, has begun dating a newly divorced man. She isn't so sure it's a good idea. "He's nice enough," she tells us, "but he just doesn't connect. It's like he's off in his own world most of the time."

Crystal agrees with the assessment. "Never date a newly divorced man," she says, "two dates and they want to marry you. Go to bed with them and they think you're practically married already."

I watch the faces of each of the women through this conversation. They've all been through the mill and they have war stories to tell about their experiences with newly divorced men as well as stories about their own divorce experiences.

"It's a crazy time after divorce," Gina says, looking out at the rain in the parking lot and the people scurrying to get inside without getting too wet. No one, it seems, owns an umbrella in Southern California. "You want to have as much fun as you can and yet you don't want to make any bad mistakes. What you end up doing is not having much fun and making bad mistakes, anyway.

John, a construction foreman is sitting with us and is newly divorced. He agrees with what's being said. "Why are men so screwy after a divorce, doc?" he asks. "I'm a pretty healthy guy and I'm feeling really crazy these days."

Most social scientists and marital counselors believe that men follow a certain pattern of behavior after a divorce. For a certain limited time, maybe two to six months, they stay away from women. Not all of them, of course, but many of them do. Some men report a feeling of relief at not having women in their lives after a divorce.

As these feelings begin to go away and loneliness and the need for intimacy set in, men either go out in flurries of dates, or they find one person and begin to date exclusively. If they date one person at this time, they put a great deal of energy into the relationship, pointing out how different this person is from ex-wives. Often the person they are involved with is not only very much like their ex-wife but, in some ways, may be far worse. Loneliness coupled with anger at ex-wives and the need to prove that they can still attract a woman drive many men to make absolutely disastrous decisions.

In California, second marriages end in divorce in almost the same numbers, 65%, as first marriages. In other parts of the country, second marriages are likely to fail at about the same rate as first marriages (40% of the time). The risk of repeated divorce goes up when: 1) The length of time of a new marriage is 15 months or less from the time of divorce; 2) there is a great age difference between spouses (more than 10 years); 3) each of the partners have financial problems; 4) the woman's ex-husband is not paying or is underpaying child support; 5) the new husband's child support payments are so high that he can't hold up his end up of the financial necessities of the marriage; 6) there are problem children who will be living at home or who occupy considerable time, expense, and energy; 7) there are unresolved substance abuse problems; 8) An ex-husband/wife or boy-friend/girlfriend is interfering in the marriage; 9) the couple have little in common; 10) the marriage is one partner's idea and the other partner has passively accepted it.

How can women avoid second and third marriages that end in divorce? The following guidelines taken from the literature on successful second and third marriages, from the marital therapists who guide people in such decisions, and from the men and women who have discussed these issues with me in the past 30 years might help.

The Rules of Re-Marriage

I. The Heart is a Lonely Hunter

If you're dating a recently divorced man, take your time getting involved emotionally. That includes not having sex until you're both ready. If you <u>do</u> find a man who is likely to be a serious person for you to date, don't make plans to marry until you've known him for a good long time. The longer you wait to make the decision to marry, the more successful it will tend to be. Consider the following example from a client who broke all of the above rules:

"I met this great looking woman in her mid-twenties. I was feeling pretty lonely and unsure of myself at the time. My divorce had been the low point in my life. I didn't think I'd ever be interested in women again until I met Nancy. Of course, I was impressed that she thought I was attractive. The sex was stupendous. It happened right away and it just got better and more addicting. It was all I could think about. Somewhere in the back of my mind I knew that Nancy had problems, bad ones, but I was in heat. And I was jealous like I've never been before. An eyebrow change and I'd begin to suspect something. I'd have fantasies about her screwing around with other guys.

"It just got so consuming that all I could think was that if I married her, she'd be mine and I wouldn't worry anymore. So I did. I hardly knew her when we got married. After a while, I started to realize that what was in the back of my mind was the fact that, other than sex, I had nothing at all in common with her. When all of this started to dawn on me, the sex, which had been so great to begin with, just started to feel like nothing special. And she <u>was</u> messing around. I'd been absolutely right to feel jealous. Guys who get involved soon after their divorces with young women and guys who mistake sex for love are in for a rude awakening. Think my first divorce was bad? My second one was a corker and she took me to the cleaners."

II. Beauty, Sex, and Real Love

As you know, men often date women because of the way they look. Frequently, the inner beauty that many women have is lost on men, particularly men who are newly divorced. This initial phase of dating attractive women is often followed by a realization that deeper emotional needs are often met by women who have other important qualities. But it takes men time to recognize this. Don't be surprised when the man who showed little interest in you immediately following a divorce shows interest in you a year or so later. Men have fantasies about who they will date after a divorce, unrealistic fantasies, of course, but before they can make good decisions, they need to play out their fantasies by dating, or trying to date, very attractive women. As one man told me who dated a beauty queen finalist after his divorce:

"It was great for my ego for the first few months. We'd go out to dinner and everyone would stare at us; at her, really. I used to think that it made me feel special because people thought I must be pretty terrific to attract such a beautiful woman. In time, though, I just got fed up with her narcissism and I stopped seeing her as beautiful. To me she was cold and unfeeling. I started to date women who were nice people, not just good looking. And you know what? The women who were nice began to look more and more beautiful the longer I knew them. What's inside of them, in their heart, comes through in time. It's pretty amazing."

Really great men, and there are all kinds of them if you look, want more than looks. They want depth, and sensitivity, and honesty. They want to be valued and appreciated. If a man is only seeing you for your looks, his feelings for you are superficial. You have other attributes like what's is in your head, heart, and soul. If they don't see that, or if they aren't interested, don't demean yourself by getting into the looks game. It's a losing proposition with men. In time, they'll find someone better looking or they'll start noticing that you weren't quite as good looking as they thought you were. If they don't care about the inside of you, they won't care about what's outside, either.

Also, don't believe that all men are exclusively interested in looks. Maybe at first, but more mature men seek partners in life, people with whom they can share and commit. Don't take yourself out of the running for older divorced men because you think that men only seek young, beautiful women. A lot of men have been hurt by beautiful women. It's the last thing in life they want.

A sign on a bus in Mexico City I recently saw said: "All beautiful women are traitors." Most men distrust beautiful women, but nice, giving, tender women, ah, now that's another story. To these women, divorced, slightly muddled, disappointed men, flock. Trust me, you have much more to offer than you think.

III. Blind Dates, Mayhem, and Stage Fright

There are many legitimate ways to meet men such as blind dates, dating services, meeting men in the workplace, and meeting men in groups sponsored by churches and synagogues. Don't ignore dates suggested by parents, in-laws, or friends. While they sometimes don't work out, these folks have your best interest at heart and often they can make excellent choices. You won't know until you go out with the person they suggest. If you go out on a blind date, meet the first time for coffee or a movie. Don't do anything elaborate. There is no experience worse than a bad date, which is also an expensive bad date. Sometimes blind dates can work out even if they seem unlikely to in the beginning. Listen to John's experience with a blind date set up by his aunt.

"Well, I knew it was going to be a disaster before I even went out on the date. What does my aunt know about my taste in women? And then the phone call. It was like talking to the wall, she was so unresponsive. But it was my aunt and I wasn't having such great success on my own, so I went out. We met at a coffee house not far away and it wasn't a great experience, but it also wasn't as bad as I thought it would be. We were both pretty nervous and we stammered a lot at first, but after a while, we had a nice conversation. Afterward, I called up my aunt to thank her and she was surprised. She said, 'I thought you'd both hate each other but your mother was putting so much pressure on me to find you a date that Judy was the only one I could think of.' It gave me a lesson in humility. When people do something nice for you, you should respect them enough to at least try and make it work. Finally, I did meet a very nice woman on a blind date my secretary arranged. It can happen. You just need to keep your faith. Now I even set folks up. It's usually a disaster, but how else is anyone going meet some-one in this day and age?"

IV. Psychomen

Don't become involved in someone's emotional or financial problems. One rea-son women become enmeshed with troubled men very early in a relationship is that they take on responsibilities they have absolutely no business assuming just to prove themselves. Women do this a lot and the consequences can be awful, as this story from a friend will show:

"I know that most people thought Ed was pretty screwy, but we had good times and I was in love with him in the beginning. But the fact is that Ed's pretty badly put together. From the moment I met him, I was doing things for him. Small things at first and then more and more until he was so dependent on me, it didn't feel like he could do anything himself. That was bad enough but then he started to blame me for being so unhappy. How was it my fault, I'd ask? He didn't know, it just was. If I did anything for him, I was taking his independence away. If I didn't do something for him, then I didn't love him. It made me crazy being around him.

"All the time I was working so hard to please Ed, he was seeing someone else. A really conniving woman who took everything he had. Here I am being criti-cized for doing too much and what he really enjoys is being abused. To me, that's the glory of the story. It should help women know not to get involved with a man's problems before you really know what he wants from you and what he will give in return for your help. Love can be a pretty screwy emotion, and troubled men can take you to the cleaners, if you let them."

V. Dangerous Men Will Rob You of the Marrow of Your Bones

Unless you want your insides torn apart, your life wrecked, your money taken from you, and your dignity thrown in the garbage can, stay away from "danger-ous men." Dangerous men are that breed of male who don't play by rules. They seem exciting at first and terrific for your ego. They prowl after vulnerable women and then they ruin their lives. Since they don't play by the rules, they can't be trusted, and they'll do things that no responsible human being would ever do to anyone. Maybe a bit of them hates women. Often they are fun to be with, terrific looking, and smart, and they take chances that can be stimulating to those of you who are a little bored with your lives. Listen to a friend's experience:

"I was maybe 10 months into living alone after my divorce and it was everything it was cracked up to be. Major lonely. I was living in Alabama at the time and all the men I went out with acted like they were from another planet. I can't quite describe it but between those twangy accents and all the adolescent behavior, it wasn't looking very good for romance.

"I met Jan through a friend. He was really handsome and fun, right from the start. Just what I needed to get back into the swing of things. And unpredictable. Some days he was so disinterested in me, it was like being with a stranger. Other days he'd talk about marriage and commitment. Every time I was with him, something really screwy happened. Major public arguments, wrecking a motel room over something, him saying another woman's name when we were making love, big surprise baskets delivered to my work so all of my co-workers would wink at me for weeks, break-ups followed by passionate get togethers, followed by breakups. It was crazy.

"One night he came to my house and stuck a knife in my shoulder. It stopped being fun right then. It was like a scene out of <u>Fatal Attraction</u>. I had to leave the area and a great job. Stay away from dangerous men. That's all I can say to any woman who's out of a marriage, feeling lonely, and on the prowl. They'll destroy you."

VI. Kids Can Make or Break a Relationship

Before you remarry someone with children, get to know them. Find out if you can live together. Have dinner together. Go to functions together. Go on a trip, perhaps. See if you get along. Children are one of the serious stressors of second marriages. A friend told me the following story about a man she had been seeing and his troubled relationship with her child:

"We went together a long time before we finally decided to try living together. I had a three old, a really lovely little girl who adored him. He never seemed very enthusiastic about her, but she still adored him. Her dad had passed away and she had seen him die. It was very traumatic for her. A man in my life made up for a lot of the trauma she'd gone through. Anyway, he moved in and it was clear he didn't want to have anything to do with her. He ignored her, never let her sit on his lap, and avoided coming home until after she was asleep. It was really awful for my child who thought that he disliked her.

"I had to keep explaining that he was very busy and that he thought about work a lot. But it bothered me and finally I ended it. He clearly didn't like my child, would never take any responsibility for her, and wanted nothing to do with her. At the same time, he was talking about adopting her. How can you explain such a thing? It seemed utterly dishonest to me to say one thing and yet do something so different. I don't think it's going to be easy to find a man who will help me raise my child."

VII. Money Is The Root of Many Relationship Problems

Be very careful about commingling money if you're thinking about re-marrying. The happiest people I know in second marriages are those who discuss money seriously before they get married. They have an agreement about to how they'll handle common bills as opposed to personal expenses, which are the sole concern of one of the spouses. Be very careful about the way money is handled in case the marriage ends in divorce. A pre-nuptial agreement is always a good idea and whether you include spouses in wills is also very important to this process. My general rule of thumb, although you may disagree, is that children under the age of 21 should be the primary beneficiaries in wills in second marriages. Spouses should not be added until the marriage is firm and children have grown. Too many marriages take place because one spouse has money. Consider the following story a good friend of mine told me:

"My husband and I got divorced. It probably wasn't the brightest thing I ever did in my life since we weren't really that unhappy. Everyone was getting divorced back then. Soon after we divorced, maybe as a form of retaliation, he got married to a very young woman. She talked him into making her the primary beneficiary in his will instead of our two children. He died eight months after they got married, probably because she was such an unpleasant and demanding bitch. Anyway, my kids got nothing. Not a cent. We're fighting it in court, but can you imagine the way I feel? A woman is married to him for eight months and she gets everything. Me and the kids, we get nothing for the 20 years we were together. It just isn't right."

VIII. Divorced, Lonely, and Vulnerable

Women who are newly divorced are considered fair game for many unscrupulous men who often believe that newly divorced women are vulnerable or they're just out for a good time. In any case, many men see divorced women as easy pickings. Be very careful whom you date after a divorce. This is no time to act out your anger at your ex-husband by sleeping around. AIDS is everything it's cracked up to be. Furthermore, men who prey on newly divorced women can harm you in many physical and emotional ways. Consider this story from one of the ladies at the coffee shop.

"Well, I admit it, I was out looking for trouble. I was pretty mad at my ex. He took some good years from me and didn't leave me anything in exchange but a lot of bills and three kids. When I got divorced, I did a lot of bar hopping and I slept around. It was fun, I gotta say, and I met some pretty jazzy guys, some of 'em a lot younger than me. Very good for the old ego.

"Jim, he comes along with his smooth ways and before I know it, he's liven with me and takin my money. I mean I was supporting him and he could be pretty mean when he had a mind to. It got so bad I was afraid to go home after work. I got the kids out of the house and just left it for good. I know him or his friends wrecked it one night. You pay for takin too many chances."

And The Ladies Have The Last Word

Janine, one of the infrequent members of the group looks over at me when I'm done talking and says, to cap off the discussion we've been having about men and divorce, "I met my husband after he was divorced about a year. All the things you said are pretty true. He was a mess, but then, so was I. I came out of a divorce that was plain awful. My husband tried to kill me. Nothing happened legally but he stalked me, threatened me, and beat me up one night. He hasn't seen the kids in four years. To avoid paying child support, he left the area and got another social security card so he can't be traced. I wasn't in a very good place to start a new relationship.

"Somehow, Jack and I just hit it off. We knew we were both pretty damaged from what happened in our marriages and the problems we had with our divorces. But we were good people who liked each other so we made an effort, a real effort. The thing is that at some point, you need to trust men. They may be a little crazy after a divorce but a lot of them are also concerned about changing and being better. That's what I can say about my experiences after my divorce. The good ones are sometimes better after a divorce. It opens their eyes up to how important love and marriage are. It takes time and a lot of hard work to make a second marriage work after a divorce, but it's worth everything to have a good marriage after a bad one."

Everybody looks outside. The sun is breaking through the gloom. It's another California day. Who knows what will happen? That's the thing about California. It beats you into the ground, sucks the life out of you, throws you around like you were a rag doll, and then it lets you start a new day with hope and energy.

All the people who meet in the coffee shop are survivors of divorce. It's awful experience, but somehow we pick ourselves up, shake the hurt from our bodies, try and be better the next time, and we get on with our lives. We weren't made to live alone but we should go about the difficult job of finding a mate with care and patience. And when we get it right, it's just about the best thing that can ever happen.

8

Gunslinger Blues: The Sad and
Lonely Life of the Divorced Man

Free, Single, And Miserable

Most divorced men do not romp through the woods having orgy after orgy. In fact, many newly divorced men are reluctant to get involved with women at all. Loneliness and sexual need drive them into relationships that are sometimes disastrous. A friend of mine describes the relationship problems he's had since his divorce as love in the war zone. It isn't a real war, he adds, it's just that every time he enters into relationships, he comes away wounded.

This war zone of relationships, this gender war we seem to be in makes many of us miserable. What do they want? I am asked of the women who, yet another time, do something just plain mean-spirited. Why can't I ever meet someone nice? asks the woman fresh from another bad experience.

Joan, a CPA in her early forties comes up to me early one morning at the coffee shop and asks if she can talk to me. She looks around to see if anyone is watching. "Can I talk to you, doc, before the other ladies come in?" I nod my head, still bleary eyed. It's dark outside and even the cooks are shaking the sleep from their eyes.

She fidgets, running her hands over the coffee cup as if the cup is ballast to keep her from tipping over. She looks down at her feet and then she begins to talk very quietly. "I started going out with this guy after my divorce. At first, he was very nice to me. He helped me not feel so lonely. But in time I noticed that he was mean to people. He'd be very obnoxious to waitresses when we went out for dinner, that sort of thing. Pretty soon, I was getting it. He couldn't find a good thing about me. He just kept saying that I was just like his ex. I got fed up and left and, boy, did I get an ear full then. Calls late at night accusing me of being a liar and of having sex with other men. Things like that. My friend Jean calls them psycho-men, they're so crazy. I don't know why doc, but I seem to attract every single crazy man out there. How do you find men you can trust?"

A very good question. This is my list of what to look for in men who you might find to be trustworthy.

Choosing Men You Can Trust

1) Men you can trust never ask you for money. Either they have their own or they are too proud to take money from you, even if they need it.

2) Men you can trust have a good working relationship with ex-wives and get along well with their children. Look for signs from the past. Men who have good relationships with ex-lovers are men who will be good to you. Men whose ex-lovers want to kill them are men to stay away from.

3) Men you can trust care about your health and welfare. They'll be there if you need them in a crunch. They'll ask about your health. If need be, they'll go with you to a doctor's appointments or offer to help in some way if you're ill. Look for signs of concern and honest efforts to help out.

4) Men you can trust respect your feelings and don't try to shape you in a certain way. The man who starts talking about the things you could do in your life if you only went back to a school, or learned certain information, or had a certain specific interest, is saying that you're not good enough now.

5) Men you can trust have planned financially for the future. They don't expect to be cared for by a woman. In fact, they find this need for dependency on a woman very unappealing. They want to be healthy and independent for as long as their health will permit. If they are dependent on you initially, it will probably increase with time.

6) Men you can trust keep promises. They don't stand you up on dates or break dates at the last moment for cockamamie reasons. If they do, it's a sign of an uncaring person who senses that he can do anything he wants to you and you won't mind.

7) Men you can trust are punctual and respect your attitudes about time. Men who are chronically late when they know it upsets you will probably not change in time. If anything, they're uncaring behavior may only get worse.

8) Men you can trust do not play head games to get you into bed. You're not an adolescent anymore and you've heard every line a man can come up with. Don't go to bed with any man until you are emotionally ready. Good men won't try to con you. They, like you, don't want intimacy until they're ready for it.

9) Men you can trust do not have wandering eyes. If they do, it just means that they're minds and bodies will probably follow their eyes.

10) When all else fails, the best predictor of future behavior is the past. If men have acted badly in the past, chances are they'll do the same in the future.

The Wise Woman's Guide To Relationships

Let's assume you now know the men to stay away from. How do you approach dating so that you'll find and keep a good man? Try these rules of relationships on and see if they work for you.

1. The First Rule of Relationships: A good relationship starts with companionship and friendship. It usually doesn't start with great sex or with romance. That may come in time, but for a relationship to be successful, there has to be a foundation. Your mother was right about this one. Listen to her advice. Don't get involved with men who make you feel like you're the greatest thing since sliced bread, particularly if you feel that way from the moment you meet. That feeling of wonder and joy is an indication that your defenses are down and that you may be super susceptible to impulses that may get you into a great deal of emotional trouble.

My daughter tells me that I'm absolutely wrong about this. She thinks that infatuation is the first step in a successful relationship. If you aren't infatuated, she asks, then how do you know there's any fire in the relationship? Good question. The answer I've given her is that there is a great deal of difference between infatuation and liking someone. When you're infatuated, your emotions are already working over-time and you're in a poor position to rationally see a man as he really is. When you like someone, you're in control of your emotions. You can proceed with the small and large steps that define how serious a relationship will become.

I don't think my daughter is moved by this reasoning but then, of course, she's only sixteen and enough infatuations in her life may make her more cautious. For you, however, mature and intelligent women that you are, beware of the loss of reason that accompanies your first few experiences after divorce with someone you like much more than you should. If you like someone right off the bat and you're feeling really out of control, take a deep breath, get some distance, and proceed with caution. Infatuation may lead to love or it may lead you down the road of very hurt feelings. Don't move too quickly when your emotions are out of control and don't let the man do it, either.

My good friend Lila tells me that most women love to be infatuated and that they won't continue to date a man unless they are. "I don't understand it in women," she says. "They seem not to learn from past experience. Every bum who makes their heart beat faster, right off the bat, that's the bum they fall for even if it always leads to trouble. And it happens again and again for a lot of women. They never seem to learn. I know women who are madly in love after one date. Mature women. And do they get hurt? Of course they do.

"You would think that after a few experiences they'd know better, but it just keeps happening. They go out with abusive, drunken creeps, but if they feel strong emotions, then look out below, they think they're in love. My god, you'd think they'd learn, wouldn't you?"

2. The Second Rule of Relationships: Men often don't like making plans months into the future when they're not giving out any signals that they're ready for a serious relationship. Keep your plans short-term at first, perhaps a week or so, until you both start talking about longer-term plans. And don't use the word love. It's better with men to talk about exclusive relationships, which mean that neither of you will date or sleep with other people. It does not necessarily mean that you are in love or that the relationship will lead to marriage. An exclusive relationship means that two mature people are doing what is necessary to see if the relationship might lead somewhere, unencumbered by the hurts and problems that come if they are dating other people at the same time.

For most mature men, the word love means something very special. Men won't use the word unless they feel deeply. Beware of men who use the word in the midst of love making. Men and women say things when they make love that may be very impulsive or unrelated to the way they really feel. Nothing said in bed is ever a substitute for what is said in the cold hard reality of two people saying good night at the end of a date.

3. The Third Rule of Relationships: If he is like the man before who broke your heart, stay as far away from him as you can. It's very true that we have a tendency to repeat mistakes and to form patterns in our relationships. Some therapists feel that our attraction to others is based on unconscious tendencies that are imprinted in our brain early in our lives. That may be true but, as adult men and women, we can be aware of patterns and attempt to change them.

One way to do this is by going out with men who are very different from those who usually attract us, just to test the waters. You may be surprised at how very pleasant an experience it can be to date men who come from different backgrounds and are very unlike the prior men in your life.

If you've been in dysfunctional relationships, be especially careful in the men you choose. Look for signs of problems such as bad tempers or extreme jealousy. Don't ignore indications of alcohol or drug abuse. Be particularly attentive to the stories men tell you about why their marriages failed. There are little gems of insight in these stories that may have meaning for you. Many men, in time, may treat you in ways similar to the ways they treated their ex-wives, so be very careful about the man who promises to treat you differently. The best predictor of the future is the past.

My friend Marjorie tells the story of the man who was about to divorce his wife of 25 years. He was dating a single friend of hers and the friend was in seventh heaven. Marjorie thought the guy was a real creep, but didn't want to interfere or hurt her friend's feelings. "He told my friend that he'd slapped his wife around some," she said "but it was only because she drove him to it. She told him that he drank too much at times, but again, it was because his wife pushed him to drink. And guess what? He did the same things to her. My friend was shocked. She couldn't understand what she had done to deserve such treatment. She hadn't done anything except to get involved with a sick and abusive guy who was out of control. What a man will do to someone else, they'll probably do to you."

4. The Fourth Rule of Relationships: No one said it was easy. Relationships are hard work. If you aren't willing to work at one, you may not be ready. At the same time, the work should have a payoff. You should see tangible results from your hard work. You'll have to define what that tangible result is, but for most of us, you should be happier with someone than you are when you're alone. If that isn't the case, it's time to consider the reasons you're in a relationship that gives you no pleasure.

Some friends of mine, in typical yuppie fashion, never quite got it right about relationships. For them, a relationship was something you toiled over like a garden. It was hard, unrewarding work. They talked about everything until it withered and died. And they were deadly serious about it. Who was going to do the shopping? It was a three month discussion. Were they spending enough time with the kids? A never-ending discussion. They'd been to EST and to marriage encounters galore. They'd been in sensitivity groups and marriage enrichment groups.

The guy was seeing someone on the side. The woman was beginning a gay relationship. It was such a mess that, when it all fell apart, the guy tried to kill his wife. The endless talk covered everything except what was really vital to the relationship: whether they cared for each other and how to make that sense of caring, grow.

5. The Fifth Rule of Relationships: Nice men, honest men, are worth a whole lot more than flashes in the pan. Men who make you feel great one day and awful the next are no one's idea of terrific people. Unless you want to be miserable much of the time (and who does?), start going out with nice men. They may be less than exciting at first, or they may not make you feel as if they are the great love of your life, but with openness and practice comes mastery. The more open you are to a range of men and the more you resolve to go out with men who are safe, the better your chances of finding the right person. They may not be the most handsome of men or the greatest lovers, but you'll come to appreciate the qualities that make them good people and you'll l be all the more happy for it.

On the other hand, inconsiderate men can wreck havoc in your life. Consider this story a friend told me not long ago. "I just came out of a bad marriage and I wasn't in a rush to get involved with anyone. My daughter and I were at Yosemite National Park having a great time when I met this fabulous looking guy in the pool. We talked a lot and agreed that I'd look him up when I came to his hometown a month later on business. I looked him up all right and that turned out to be the worst mistake of my life.

"We got involved sexually pretty fast. It was incredible sex for me, considering how bad sex had been with my ex. He was very tender and loving while we made love, but pretty aloof out of bed. Later, when I confronted him, this is maybe three months after our long distance relationship began, he told me that he had a form of cancer and that he was about to go through a number of medical procedures. Of course by then I was in love with him and before I knew it, I was flying a thousand miles to be with him whenever he felt down or scared. He started to talk about marriage and all sorts of things that led me to believe that he was in love with me.

"Imagine how I felt when it became clear that he was seeing someone else and had been all the time we were dating. He denied it all over the place, but it was obvious to me because of the secret phone calls he'd take in the bedroom for an hour or more and the far away looks he'd get. For six months I ran like a crazy woman all over the country to be with him.

"It didn't dawn on me until later that it was pretty damn mean and dishonest of him not to tell me about his cancer when we first met. When I broke it off, it felt like I was losing my sanity. I felt guilty that I'd left him while he was still ill, and angry that I'd gotten involved with him in the first place. I used to have dreams about him. He was always a vampire in my dreams and I was always having my blood sucked out of me. That's the way I remember him. As a vampire. It's made me very careful with men ever since."

6. The Sixth Rule of Relationships: Be receptive to a man but protect yourself at the same time. Let your feelings for the person slowly grow and build. Someone said that love knows not good nor bad but goes where the wild heart leads. If you believe that, as a colleague once told me, you may be in for the surprise of your life.

"I believe in being conservative," my colleague told me over lunch a few years ago. "No one you get involved with too fast is ever going to last. It's got to be slow or it won't work. Older people like us have to be careful.

"I was sort of floundering in life. I'd been divorced for ten years with no prospects in sight. My career was stuck in place and I was feeling bored with life. I met this lady in my class. It's a no-no, of course, but it happened. She worshipped me. Couldn't say enough good things about me. The sex was great. I was as happy as a pig in slop.

"The class stopped and she was still talking about the class and about me as if I was still the teacher. I'd remind her that I wasn't the teacher anymore, but sometimes she'd make a mistake and call me Doctor Jones instead of my first name. We were having sex by then and in the middle of love making she'd call me Doctor Jones. It was pretty hurtful.

"It didn't last, needless to say, but it did teach me a lesson about jumping head first into a relationship with someone I hardly knew. By the way, she filed a sexual harassment grievance against me when we broke up. I went through hell for six months, and I almost lost my nice tenured job. You live and you learn, but this lesson I learned real well. Don't jump into a relationship until you know the person really well."

7. The Seventh Rule of Relationships: We all go through periods when we can't seem to meet anyone. The poet Richard Brautigan likened this time to being a fly on a piece of meat in a greasy spoon in the middle of summer and not being able to attract a fly of the opposite sex. These slow periods in our lives can be maddening. You try and ride them out but, inevitably, whatever you do seems to either make no difference or it makes matters worse. Fritz Perls once said that in times like this we shouldn't try and push the river but instead, we ought to go with the flow. Easy for him to say, particularly if you're lonely, but good advice, anyway.

Whatever you do, remember Glicken's seventh rule of relationships: for everyone of us, someone is out their to form a pair, a match. Listen to my friend Ellen on the subject:

"I always thought that I was pretty unattractive, from the first time I dated to the present. It's just a fact. I never thought that I could attract anyone and yet men have passed through my life in a steady stream. I never thought anyone great would enter my life but I have one of the all time great husbands. It really surprises me when handsome men seem interested in me. I can't imagine why. I think it's good luck or some quality I'm missing, but then I look in the mirror and I see an overweight, middle aged woman whose looks have been consistently bad since birth. I know I shouldn't describe myself that way, but it's the truth.

"I believe that most women don't learn to see themselves as men see them. I think that if they did, they'd be more keyed into what men find attractive. I think men find a woman's voice, intellect, and brains more attractive than most women think. All I know is that some great men have seen something in me that I don't see in my self. It's very curious."

The Single Life

I know a number of men who are much happier being single than being married. They report that the freedom they experience as single men is liberating and that life is easy. But I also know men who are unhappy with single life and frankly, I think that most older men, men who have been married and have children, feel that single life is unnatural and lonely.

Singles dating in America can be tough. To begin with, how do we meet eligible people? When we do meet them, how do we know that they're alright emotionally and, in this day and age of AIDS, physically healthy? Who is there to be your guide through the muddied waters of single life?

And the answer is, usually no one. Like all of us who end relationships in divorce or separation, we've often haven't been single in a very long time. It doesn't feel right to be single. We aren't ready for it emotionally or prepared for the changes in dating behaviors since we were single last.

In earlier times, the matchmakers and the wise men and women of the community helped single people meet suitable spouses. Unfortunately, that's often no longer the case. Friends are afraid to line us up because a bad date can lead to hard feelings. Tough as it is to meet nice people, there are strategies that you might use to meet suitable people.

The best strategy I know is to find men you like in the social contacts we all have and let them know that you're available. Be cool about it, and, of course, not everyone is going to want to go out for reasons that have nothing to do with you necessarily. Like women, men may not be in a good place to date. They may be getting over another relationship or they may not want to complicate their lives by dating. Rejection isn't fun, but it happens. Don't personalize it.

My second suggestion to meet nice eligible men is to be where the men are. Contrary to popular belief, that is not in bars. The best place to look for men are the universities and colleges in your community where male students, staff, and faculty are in abundance. Take a course or two, go to the student union, attend workshops and special events. The men there are more likely to be serious, yet interesting, and are often unattached.

My third suggestion is to ask singles friends to a potluck dinner with the understanding that each person will bring another friend of the opposite sex who is unattached and is interested in meeting new people. Everyone brings something for the dinner. The experience isn't embarrassing or difficult because you know at least a few of the people. Make sure that the seating arrangement keeps people who know each other separated so that guests might interact with people they don't know.

Finally, you meet men everyday. In the supermarket, on the bus, at work, at church, you name it. Men are around who are looking for nice, competent, mature, safe relationships. Be assertive. Start conversations, reach out to them in ways that aren't threatening and you'll be surprised how happy they might be for your attention.

And the Ladies Have the Last Word

We file out of the coffee shop and head for our respective jobs. Jo Ann, a woman who works in one of the departments at my university walks up to me and thanks me for these early morning meetings. "Dr. Glicken," she says, "I don't think you know how much the women enjoy our meetings. Some of them have made some terrible mistakes in their lives but they hang in there and they stay optimistic. It's pretty amazing, really, and to have a man who can appreciate their hard work, that's really something. Thank you."

I watch Jo Ann drive off toward work and wonder how women do it. The responsibilities for children, the money problems, tough, unrewarding job. It makes me hopeful about the future and driving to work, I notice the women taking their children to school while doing their makeup and having their coffee, all at the same time. Amazing, I think, and I'm filled with a feeling of great joy thinking that I'll see many of these same women in a day or two and that their resilience will again, astonish me.

9

I'm All Grown Up Now but I Still Feel Like a Kid: Men and Their Parents

I'm sitting alone at the coffee shop one foggy morning during the period in Southern California known as June gloom. It's cold and damp outside and it feels good to be inside the warm and dry coffee shop. Across the aisle from me four men are having a prayer meeting. This is not unusual and I see many young Christian men in the coffee shop meeting early before work, their Bibles out, reciting chapters related to some issue of importance in the lives of one or more of the men.

Today I hear them recite the 23rd psalm of King David. One of the men is crying. His father has passed away and I overhear the things he says about his father after the psalm is read. He is full of confused feelings about his father, he explains to the men at the table. His father was a difficult man and he doesn't know how to deal with his recent death.

"He was not a Christian," the man says. "He didn't have a good heart and he didn't love his children. He was not right with God when he died, and he was not right with his children. We all harbor ill will for him even now that he is dead."

The group leader tries to comfort him but the young man is disconsolate and morose. He is sure, he tells the assembled men that his father will cast a shadow on his life for a very long time to come. I feel sorry for him because he has accurately identified the impact of his father's death. The journey he must take to cope with the effect his father had on him will not be easy.

The death of a parent is an event that often throws people into a tailspin. But when a man loses his father, and when the relationship between father and son has been strained, the psychological impact can be severe. Men look to their fathers for approval. When fathers are no longer present, where do men go to for feedback about their lives? In no small way, the death of a father forces men, even middle age men, to recognize that they are now adults.

When my father died, it was as if the ballast I carried to keep me from sinking slowly, seeped out of me. My mother had died 16 months earlier and now both of my parents <u>and</u> my marriage were dead. To cope with it all, I did what many man do. I went into a depression which I covered up with bravado, bluster, and alcohol. In reality, I was angry at my father for dying before I had a chance to really tell him why I disliked him so and for being a lousy father and husband and the most self-centered person I had ever known. Most of all, I was angry at him for doing the cruel things to his family that almost destroyed us.

My father and I were at war. It began so early in life that I can hardly remember when it started, or why. I suppose it began over his immigrant view of the world. He had seen life in the Russian Ghetto during the Czar. He understood that Jews were eternally at risk. He graced my life with daily assaults on my senses about the jeopardy we were in if I didn't toe the line…his line. These messages about how to survive in a hostile world helped me later in life to deal with the many hardships and problems, which always present themselves along the way. But in those early years after World War II, I wanted to be like everyone else. I didn't want to think of myself as an immigrant kid or to think of the treachery and danger lurking around the corner because I was Jewish and poor.

The more we fought and the higher the stakes, the better I got at the little insults, the put downs that offended him the most. Nothing was sacred. His accent, his lack of money, his blue collar job on the railroad. Everything was fair game in this war of wills we were fighting.

And yet, I was intensely proud of him as, I think from discussions I have had with my family after his death, he was proud of me. He kept our family together when my mother's medical bills outstripped his income by two or three times. He was involved in the labor movement and helped organize the part of rural, conservative America I grew up in, surely not an easy thing for an immigrant Jew in a place without other Jewish people. He had a hunger for life and introduced me to opera and good literature, to plays, to sports and nothing ever since has excited me more than going to the movies with him and listening to him tell me the way some blockbuster movie was made. It was all spectacular and wonderful as seen through his eyes.

He was proud in his soul of being an American. The word "America" thrilled him. He saw America as the lucky place for his family where a Jew could succeed. And he hated anyone who said anything bad about the country. I heard stories from cronies of his after he died of times when he had physically fought with a communist or an anarchist trying to impede the labor movement in America after the First World War. My friends adored him, for he had the gift of the gab and he could make any time special when my friends came to our little house.

But when he died, I could only think of the many hurts, the moments of pain between us, and it began to destroy me. I took to having long arguments with him in my mind about past hurts as I showered or drove to work. His voice was with me when I slept. I thought I saw him several times at work walking through a crowd, shaking his head at me. For months after his death we fought the fights I hadn't been able to resolve when he was alive.

There is no war more desperate or bloody than the war between a dead father and his son. It is a war for mastery of the spirit, for the right to be a man, for the ritual rights of passage that allow a child to become an adult.

I didn't master the anger I was feeling for my father easily. It took work and it took time, for the need to stay a child, to deny my manhood and remain a boy was very powerful. I finally sought help in the form of therapy, but what brilliant therapy. Therapy done by geniuses that took me from childhood, to adolescence, to adulthood in fifteen minutes. When it was over, I walked a country road and marveled that there could be such beauty in the world, beauty I hadn't seen before. I felt my father's loss and I grieved for him as I had failed to do when he died.

Several years later, at a national conference, I gave one of the early papers on men and our issues. My 12 year old daughter Amy sat in the audience. I told the audience that I would never be as successful as my father had been, nor would I achieve at the same level he had. I said these things lovingly and without question. My father was a remarkable man, an admirable man. He was also a difficult and thoughtless man who could be cruel beyond measure. But in my mind today, as I look back and collect my memories, he is also a heroic man for the many struggles he overcame, for keeping our family together, for being a man of conviction in his work, and for being socially responsible.

You take the good and the bad and you tally it all up. My dad, like many fathers, was a flawed man full of blazing contradictions and terrible inconsistencies. He could be wonderful one minute and then he could be just plain mean the next. I prefer to remember him as a special man who did good things, whose children made it, who taught us to live life to its fullest.

I can put the bad parts of him aside and focus on the good he did. I remember the specialness, I think of the complexity of his personality, and it makes me think more positively of him and of myself. I am a part of him and these special memories of him make me feel much better about myself.

Whose View of Dad Do Men Buy?

I had a wonderful African American student by the name of Arthur Clark. Art is as much my friend now as he was my student. We play racquetball together and work out in the gym when I need help keeping in shape. Art is a former football player and in such great shape that he exudes health.

Some years ago, Art took a course from me in crisis intervention. He was testing the waters to further his career, not sure if he wanted to be in education as he currently was or if the larger arenas of life such as public administration and policy work were more suited to him.

As is my practice whenever I teach a class, I asked for a volunteer to role play the type of therapy I do. I'm very active in my therapy. Arthur asked to role-play a problem he was having with his father. In Arthur's opinion, his father was an alcoholic. I did what one would normally do. I asked Arthur on what he based this judgment. He said, "My father drinks all day long and I'm afraid that he won't be alive when I need him the most."

"All day long?" I asked.

"Pretty much," Arthur responded.

"How many drinks would that be?" I wondered.

Arthur shook his head. "I don't really know," he said, "I never counted."

"But you're sure that he's an alcoholic," I asked.

Arthur just sat staring at me. No one had ever questioned this view of his father. It just was a fact in his mind. His father drank too much. So, as is typical of the way I work, I asked Arthur to role play a confrontation with his dad. He was to tell his dad that he worried about his drinking and that he was afraid that his father wouldn't be alive when Arthur needed him most. Mind you, this was all done in front of a class of 25 other students. Arthur said the following:

"Dad, I worry that you drink too much and that your health will suffer. I want you to be part of my life, to see me when I'm successful in life, to see my kids grow up. I don't want you to die early like so many black men."

I listened to what Arthur had said throughout his discussion about his father and I took a chance. In therapy you have little to go on other than your intuition and your empathic understanding of the human condition. So I said the following to Art, but I said it playing the role of his father.

"Arthur (I used his formal name because I was convinced that his father used it and that it would have more clout in the role play), Arthur where did you get this idea that I drink too much? I worked for 40 years. I went to work everyday. I provided for everyone. We had a good life. I'm retired now, Arthur, and I have a nip or two with the boys, with my friends. Does that make me an alcoholic?"

Art's head snapped back, literally. He looked at me for a long time and then he said, "But that's what mom says about you, that you drink too much."

In the role play I leaned over and touched Arthur on the arm and then I said, "But Arthur, your mom is a very religious woman. Any drink is too much for her, you know that. Why shouldn't I enjoy these retired years and have some fun? And if I take a drink or two, so what? I'm a healthy man, I've worked hard, and I'm not irresponsible. Aren't I entitled to enjoying these years after working so hard? You have your dad alive and well. There aren't many Black sons who can say that. Why not enjoy me instead of criticizing me?"

I looked over at Arthur and tears were coming out of his eyes. Like most men who have been given permission to see their fathers as human beings, he was overwhelmed by the experience. It was liberating not to carry the burden of a father who had somehow failed his son.

When Arthur composed himself, he turned to the class and said that no one had ever given him the opportunity to talk about these things. He thought it wasn't masculine to discuss problems. Now he knew how wrong that was and that it was clear he wanted to be in social work, if this was what we did to help people. "How many Black youth would benefit from a similar discussion?" he asked the class. And then he answered his own question. "All of them," he said, "all of us."

Arthur was admitted into the MSW Program I taught in. He was the winner of many awards and is moving on to get his doctorate. He hasn't decided where, but since I mentor him, it will be somewhere high level where his career will be as good and as successful as I know it can be.

Six months after that initial interaction with Arthur, he asked me if we could go out to dinner at a new Cajun restaurant in the area close to where I live. He wanted me to meet his father.

The night stands out in my mind. It was such great fun because, much as I had guessed, his father was a man of great joy. A cut up and a story teller, charismatic and kind. His father made me think of my own father who now, passed away, would have been like Arthur's father. I never told this to Arthur but that night was like being with my own father at a point in time when I would have appreciated him all the more for his ability to make an ordinary time so much fun.

Arthur has gone back to Louisiana with his dad to meet relatives and to discover his roots. He sees his father often and they share in the ways adult men can share when the curtain has been lifted. Arthur now sees his dad as a man with flaws and with goodness, a complex person too complicated to easily categorize. And it has been freeing for him.

We were having coffee one afternoon after seeing a movie, and Arthur reminded me of the time in class when he was able to work out some issues about his dad. He said the words of an old spiritual to me to describe how he felt. He said to me, "Free at last. Lord all mighty, thank God, I'm free at last."

Were it always so easy, of course. Were every man with problems so easy to free up. And yet, there is something about this experience that I see repeated, again and again, in the daily contacts I have with men. Most of the men I know carry deeply ambivalent views of their fathers. Most of the men I know have poor memories of their dads. Often those memories come from other people. The abandoned wife tells her son the stories of the father wrapped up in her particular anguish and disappointment. The son never hears a more well balanced view of his father. He never knows what problems, what demons his father had to contend with, or the more complete reasons for the father's behavior. No man who leaves a family fails to feel great shame.

The son doesn't hear the father's side. In time, the son cannot hear the father's side even if the father tries a reconciliation with his son. By then, his anger is too great and too much damage has been done.

Am I forgiving the behavior of men who abuse wives, abandon families, or do the many cruel and hurtful things that men sometimes do? Of course not. I am saying that boys need balanced views of their fathers, but almost never get them. In time, the loathing they feel for their fathers becomes the self-loathing they feel for themselves. Boys can never think well of themselves if the father who helped create them abandons, abuses, or ignores his children and spouse.

I make this issue of seeing the father accurately an important part of my work with men. A balanced view of fathers goes a long way toward helping men not to feel such anger at fathers. Seeing a father as a human being full of frailties, knowing the circumstances surrounding a father's behavior, understanding that all behavior operates in some purposeful way helps men feel better about their fathers and about themselves. I think the following story by a workman who came to fix my house one day illustrates what happens to men when memories are distorted:

"My dad left us when I was about ten. I don't remember much about him but my mother said he was a real son of a bitch and that he used to beat up on her and on us a lot because he was into the booze. Funny, but I don't remember any of that. Neither does my sister. For twenty years I had this anger in me over what he did. I'd listen to my mom, watch her as she got old and alone, think that he was responsible for how poor we were, and just hate the hell out of him for what he did. I mean, how to do you just up and leave a family?

"So anyway, I get married and about five years into the marriage, damned if I didn't do the same thing. I'm not proud of myself, mind you, but it happens. My wife was just dumping on me all of the time. Nothing I did was good enough. From morning to night all I ever heard was how bad I was. I had my fill of it and, one day, I just took off.

"Well, it got me to thinking about my dad and I started looking for him. I found him through the V.A. It wasn't easy, but finally, I got his address and phone number. He was living up in Bakersfield, an easy drive. Figured I'd drive up and back in the same day. Thought I'd see him, tell him off, and leave. I ended up staying three days. He was happy to see me. Made me promise to go back to my wife. Said he'd tried going back to my mom a number of times but she wouldn't let him and that he'd written us or called me and my sister, but she stopped the letters. Said he always felt guilty about leaving, but he was just a young man and not very good at talking things through. Mentioned the stuff that my mom was doing to him, her nagging and her putting him down so he didn't feel like a man anymore. It sounded pretty familiar. Said he never drank, never abused anyone.

"I go back home and confront my mom. She admits to me that he was telling the truth, but that her feelings were hurt so she made up the story. Says he paid child support for a long time. I asked how she could do such a thing, that it had a bad affect on me for a long time. She shrugs her shoulder. Men are all shits, she says. What difference does it make?

"Well, it made a difference to me, I said, and I'm gonna get to know him, which is what I did. He's no perfect man, but he's a good man and he's someone I feel proud to call my father. We do a lot of stuff together now. We like the same things, how about that? I see him every week or two. He's almost ready to retire and he may move down here to be closer, or my wife and I may move up there. It depends on where the work is. My dad just opened a trust fund for my daughter so she could go to college. Wants me to go too. Says he thinks I'm smart enough and that he's gonna take some courses. Never too old to learn, he says. Goes to show you how wrong you can be when you listen to someone else tell you about your dad. I should have found out for myself a lot sooner. It would have saved me from being so mad all these years. I bet there are a lot of men out there who have the same problem."

I'll bet he's right. In fact, one of my colleagues shared a story with me about his dad that shows how many men begin to redefine their fathers as they mature in life. "My brother and I were running wild after my old men left us. Why we didn't end up in jail is beyond me. My mother became an alcoholic after he left. Went through men like they were going out of style. Married six times before I left high school. I hated the son of a bitch for what he did to us.

"One day I was back from the service visiting my mom. We couldn't find the guy she was living with at the time. We went looking for him and found him in the barn where he'd hung himself. There he was, twisting in the wind, dead as hell. My mom just looks at him and says to us, 'Another son of a bitch bites the dust.' That's what she said to me and my brother. We both looked at her. I think we were thinking the same thing at the same time.

"My brother went looking for my dad and found him in some nursing home over in Napa where he'd gone to live after he left my mom. Says my mom was the most difficult woman he'd ever known, that she was drinking before he left, and that she was going through men right and left. We couldn't believe him because we thought that he was making it up to make himself look good, but he told us to make a few phone calls to people who knew them when they were still together, and gave us some names, and we called. It was an eye opener. He was telling the truth.

"You don't go from hating the guy who left you to loving him, but I feel better about myself now. I thought he left us because he hated me and my brother. It didn't occur to me that it was all about my mom. To me, she was a saint for having kept us together after he left. I could never see her doing anything wrong to anyone. It sounds strange, given the drinking and all the men, but that's the way I felt. I still do, for that matter. I see my dad once in a while. We don't have much to say to each other. I see him out of respect and to remind myself that you need to have a relationship with your dad, even if it isn't a good one."

Even the fighter, George Forman, believes that not knowing about your father puts children in a terrible rage. He didn't find out about his father until he was 26 and his father had long ago passed away. "I had this awful anger in me," he says. "Not knowing anything about my father was part of the reason. He never knew me, either. It's a terrible shame. There is rage in the boy who doesn't know anything about his dad. He doesn't know where he comes from, in a way. His dad doesn't know anything about him. It's got to have a bad affect. It did on me. I wanted to hurt people because of the teasing I got because I didn't know who my father was."

Are Mothers As Important As Fathers To Men?

Women are terribly important to the development of boys. Boys learn from their mothers and from the important women in their lives to control their more aggressive impulses. Mothers teach boys to be more caring and moderate in their behavior. They also teach boys about nurturing and love. And yet, boys who grow up in female dominated homes are often more angry and more in need of proving themselves. When men are absent, moderating messages fail to be reinforced by men and are frequently challenged by boys. Consider the following story told to me by a client many years ago when I was working in corrections in Minnesota. This was a recently paroled, but very violent young man whose prior history suggested that he would very likely to get into serious trouble after leaving prison.

"I love my ma. She kept the family together when my dad died in Korea. She was a kind person, but she could never understand that we needed to walk the streets. On the streets you need to be tough, to make people respect you. She'd tell us to run when someone was after us or to let them have our lunch or some money rather than risk being hurt. No way would that happen. If it did, we'd never be able to walk the streets without someone knowing that we was chicken.

"I'd tell her this and she'd shake her head. No, she'd say, it's not the right way. You'll get into trouble that way. What did my ma know about trouble? She thought the street was the place you met neighbors and tipped your hat and said, "Howdy do." She didn't know anything about the real life of any guy, and how everybody challenges you and how you've got to be prepared.

"Sure I got into trouble. Sure I coulda run. Sure I'd probably not be in the joint if I did. But you gotta live with yourself, don't ya? No man can live with himself if he thinks that running will solve any problems."

Contrast that with another felon I worked with at the same time who came from an intact home, wasn't violent, and had done some good work in prison to change his thinking about getting into trouble. "Yeah, my dad was down last week. I got into some trouble in the joint and he was pissed at me. I'm almost ready to be released and here I mess it up. My dad, he gives straight common sense messages. I listen to him more and more now. He was in the joint when he was a kid and he thinks it's time for me to grow up and start making it. My ma says the same thing but my dad's been here. Something about that makes me listen to him more, to think he knows what he's talking about. I think it'll work this time when I'm out of the joint. My dad says he's gonna be watching me real close for signs of slipping. When I do, he'll come down on me real hard. I hope he does. I need it I think."

It isn't a very complicated notion. Boys learn from their parents. If there are problems in the marriage, it affects children. When men leave homes or are drunk or abusive, naturally, everyone has a negative view of the father. The more this negative view of father influences a boy, the angrier he will be. The more he thinks of his father as a bad person, the more the son will see himself, his off spring, in the same way. Try and be fair to the memories of your boys' father. It may be difficult, particularly if he was an unfeeling, abusive and altogether awful man. But as a boy feels about his dad, in time, that's the way he will feel about himself.

Women help moderate boys. You teach boys values and to be civil instead of the little monsters their genes tell them to be. As you often teach them about being a man. Your message about what it means to be a man may be the only message he ever gets if no man is present in a boy's life. For those of you who are single and have an ex-husband who has abandoned his kids, try and have another man do some of the modeling for your sons. That man might be a brother, or a friend, or a Big Brother. Boys need good male role models. More than girls, who often use many outside influences to define themselves, boys use a few important men to learn about being men. If there are no good men to do the modeling, they will use the bad models provided by the troubled boys they meet on the streets and in gangs.

10

Men with the Right Stuff:
Successful Fathers

Whenever my daughter comes to visit, we go to the coffee shop some mornings for breakfast. The men and women I speak to glance over at us, wondering I suppose, how an academic and a guy who gets up so early in the morning can possibly have such a young daughter. You'd be amazed at how people often think that professors are too one dimensional to have children.

From time to time, they mozzy over and greet us or tell me how pretty and nice my daughter is. She flushes with embarrassment, but my daughter knows me well and understands that I talk to people wherever I go.

Crystal comes over and gives us the paper she's just read to save me the cost of buying another one. "Hi, kid, she says to Amy, my daughter. "You've got a great dad there, kiddo. Doesn't know a hell of a lot about women, but he's trying."

Amy greets that statement with a laugh. "I've been telling him the same thing," she says.

"I think I like this child, doc," Crystal tells me and shoots me another wink that makes me go weak in the knees.

When she leaves, Amy says, "Who's that, dad?"

And I explain to her that sometimes the men and the women in the coffee shop talk to me and that Crystal joins us from time to time. Amy nods her head. She's seen it before and goes back to her omelet with a grin on her face.

"What's so funny?" I ask.

"You, dad, you."

I glance down at an article I've been reading about fathers and their children and then back at my daughter. She is everything I ever asked God for in a child. She's funny, and wise, and athletic, and smart. But would she have been so nice had she been a boy, I wonder? Would I have been as good a father?

I look back at the article I've been reading about boys and fathers. The article is by Michael Segell (Esquire, March 1995, p. 121) and I read it to Amy for her reaction. It says, "What does a son learn from his father? Simply: Whether to love women or to hate them. Whether to take pride in his work, or shrink shamefully from creative endeavor. Whether to feel comfortable and productive in the industrious world of men, or weak, insecure, alone, terrified of failure. Whether to love his children or to merely envy them.

"And what does a father learn from his son? Whether he is capable of warmth and nurturing, or fearful of intimacy. Whether he is a generous teacher and mentor, or a narcissist and authoritarian. Whether he is manful enough to foster within his child discipline, morality, and reliability, or abdicates such responsibility, with profoundly dire results, to women or to the child himself. A father transmits to his son his vision of what it means to be a man. A son teaches his father humility."

Amy agrees entirely with what I've just read. "I know lots of boys who aren't very nice to girls and I'll bet everyone of them has problems with their fathers. But the nice guys in school, they're the ones who like their fathers. But it's the same thing for girls, dad. Girls learn a lot from their dads about men. If they don't get along with their fathers, they miss out on a lot of information about men, and it shows in the way they act around boys."

"What do you mean?" I ask.

"Well, let's take Jean (a girl she sometimes talks about). Jean just got pregnant by her boyfriend and her dad kicked her out of the house. But her dad was so mean to Jean and to all the other kids, you knew she'd have to find affection somewhere else. And she did, and now she has a child and she's still a kid herself."

"What does that have to do with her dad?" I ask. "She has a mom who could have given her more self-esteem and attention to make up for her dad."

"Yeah," Amy says, pausing for a moment, "but she loved her dad the most. He was the one she cared about when she was little. And then somewhere he changed and she felt hurt and rejected. I think dads are really important to their daughters. I know that you are," she says, and goes back to her omelet without further comment.

I think about this for a while. The fact is that I know many men who do well as parents, as well, perhaps, as women in their roles as mothers. Endless examples of men who are concerned and caring fathers exist. Growing numbers of men are the sole or primary parent to their children. Increasing numbers of men challenge the right of women to have custody of children after a divorce, a right that is generally reinforced by beliefs in our society that women are always the better parent, regardless of fact. Many men take their visitation responsibilities seriously and work hard to be with their children even when distance and expense are issues of concern.

This is not to suggest that painfully bad examples of men don't exist. Of the 2,500,000 parents who abandon children each year, 90% are men. In 1992, state governments collected child support payments from only 832,000, or 12% of the 6.8 million absent parents (mostly men) whose children received Aid to Families With Dependent Children, leaving the remainder of the bill to be footed by tax-payers (Los Angeles Times, April 17, 1994, p.14). It should be remembered, however, that many of these men are permanently out of work, in jail, or at very low paying jobs. Still, the figures point to a massive problem among many fathers of denial of responsibility to children to maintain their support.

But these examples are not the majority of men. The men who are good in their roles should not suffer by being lumped together with the violent and abusive men who now seem to characterize all men in the media and in the popular consciousness. As an example of the way men feel about the popular belief that men are poor fathers, an L.A. Times interview with Ronald Bass on the stereotyping of fathers notes (April 18, 1994) said that:

> They put fathers in one big pot and stereotype us. This becomes the gender problem of men against women and fails to address the best interests of the child…When women break court orders, they aren't punished. For instance, when it's your day to see the child and she refuses, you have to drag her back to court and the judge invariably says, "Don't do it again, ma'am." Typically, there is no penalty for cutting the father out, so the mother repeats the pattern at will. (P.B7)

The Real Work of Fathers

Another time, it's spring break and Amy and I are meeting in New Mexico for a four day holiday. It's a short flight for me from Southern California. My daughter has come all the way from Iowa. This long distance visitation scheme has become the norm for us. We didn't sit down and decide that we would see one another every six weeks or so, but for the past eight years, we have done just that. I never think about the expense of these long distance visits. It seems irrelevant. I'll work a little harder and make a few extra dollars to pay for these trips. Not all men are so lucky or can so easily afford so many trips, of course.

These regular trips of ours are trips of discovery and joy. We talk, we share, we find out the things about our lives that are difficult to know over the phone. It takes a special ex-wife to allow this arrangement and my ex-wife has been won-derful. I see my daughter every six weeks or so, and during Thanksgiving and Christmas and for two months in the summer. This summer we'll go to Mexico and my daughter will help me administratively as I teach a course on Latino issues in Cuernavaca, Mexico. This desire to be together seems natural now to me but, at first, having my daughter fly to see me in California scared me. It didn't scare my daughter who thought that it was a great adventure.

I don't know that I'm a great father or that anyone will write a book about me. But I'm a good father and I care about my daughter. I resent the implication that I am the exception. All around me in the airports of America, I see divorced fathers with their children. We get little recognition for our concern. Perhaps we could do better. Who couldn't? But we try and, in our way, we add to the lives of our children and to our own inner lives. Our children make us feel alive and vital when often our work lives and our personal lives give us very little solace.

Many of us have been at the births of our children. We learned to change dia-pers along with our wives. We cooked, and washed, and sewed for our kids. We care for our children when our wives work. If we separate or divorce, we care for our children in all the ways a mother would care for a child.

I toilet trained my daughter during a period of separation from my wife when we shared time with my daughter cross-country. I had my daughter for a month and then my wife would have her a month. This went on between ages 1 and 3. I weaned my daughter from her bottle and introduced her to panties instead of diapers. No one trained me in these functions. They were taught to me by extraordinary baby sitters and by friends, and they were tested out in the labora-tory of the day to day life with a child.

I would resent anyone saying that there aren't others of us out there who do the same things I did with my daughter. The working men of America do these tasks everyday. We would rail at the notion that all men shirk from their respon-sibilities to children.

And yet a depressing number of men do little with their children. They leave the care of children entirely to wives and girlfriends. Many see children as not much more than the end results of their virility. When they separate or divorce, the children they helped conceive are like excess baggage to be dumped at the first opportunity. Half of the divorced men in America fail to pay child support. A depressingly high number fail to visit children, or they visit only occasionally. Their children go from loving them, to resenting them, to hating them. Aban-donment is never an act of grace.

These fathers spoil the lives of children and bring their wives into immediate poverty. They throw children away as if the act of conception were some sort of biological joke to them. My colleagues in the welfare departments of America tell me that all too many of these fathers have less than a clue about how many children they have fathered. When told to pay child support for a child they hardly know or don't know at all, they prance and strut and threaten. Ultimately, they deny parenthood no matter how clear the proof may be.

These are the men who use women and children, who put their needs above those of the people they should care about. One can only guess at their inner lives and wonder how bankrupt the human condition can get. Unfortunately, these men contribute to the national view of men as dead-beats. Dead-beat fathers. The word describes the men in America who abandon children and wives. These are the men who will never have a reunification with children or learn to view their children as competent and kind people who go on in their lives and contribute to society.

Ultimately, these men feel remorse and wish to reunite with their children. But by then, the damage has been done and the urge to reunite with parents is lost on the children who have had to bare the indignity of explaining to the world that their father abandoned them for no particular reason that they, or that anyone else can explain.

I have a wonderful student whose father abandoned him when he was too young to remember. A remarkable mother, with the help of extended family, raised my student to be the special person he is now. Consider what he has to say about fathers who abandon their children: "I never think about him. Well, once in a while when I'm feeling vulnerable and hurt I think about him as some wino in the alley sleeping on a cardboard box, or maybe he's in jail. In my mind he's been paid back for what he did to my mom and my sister and me. He's some diseased person, someone with sores all over his body. Maybe he has leprosy. I know I never want to meet him unless it's in some dark alley where I can do to him what he did to us. Beat him up until he has no spirit left. That's what I think about someone who'd leave a wife and small kids to fend for themselves without ever calling, or writing, or sending money. What kind of person would do that? In my mind, a monster, that's who."

Teaching Men To Be Good Fathers

When you live two thousand miles away from your child, it seems as if every day you're away from your child is a day in which they change in ways that are very subtle. It hurts to see the small changes and to know that you haven't been there for her. But as much as I love my daughter and miss her, I also know that she will grow in ways that do not always include me. I prepare myself for the hurt that is a part of the process of becoming a person apart from your parent.

Many men and women live their lives through their children. They put aside relationships or special trips with friends to be with their children. This act of loyalty to children is something children reward us for with unconditional love and loyalty. It makes us feel wonderful to have a captive audience who loves us.

And then, at a time when we are least able to understand it, children become their own people. They no longer need us as they did when they were smaller. And the love we gave them, the time and the energy we put into their lives while our lives were empty of adult love and affection, are suddenly without payback. Not a few men and women feel violated by the disloyalty of children at this time in their lives. All of a sudden the people we put our guts into caring for could positively care less about us. It hurts, if that word comes close to the pain many of us feel.

I know men and women whose children are insensitive to the fears we all have about serious illnesses. I've spoken to people whose children don't visit them in the hospital when they have surgeries, or who haven't the time to discuss personal matters. When this happens, something precious dies inside of us.

What should we do about the children of America who take so much from us but give so little in return? I have some ideas, but the best idea begins with a belief that we should never completely put aside our own needs for the needs of others. Children's needs never supersede ours. I'm around many people who think that their lives end when children enter the scene. That is never the case. Being a good parent means hours of hard work everyday. But at the same time, our lives needn't end and our personal needs shouldn't go away.

With this in mind, what are the principles of being good parents that you can share with your husband, future husband or serious partner to make him as good a father as he can be? And further, what are the principles of being a good parent that will result in children who are kind, thoughtful, loving and con-cerned—about us, their parents, and about others? Here are the ones I think are the most important.

1) To have children who care about us, you must first teach children their responsibility to parents. I believe that to have concerned and respectful children, you must teach children that they have obligations to parents which include being respectful and possibly caring for them when they are unable to care for themselves. We often think that when parents are very good to children, that

children will reciprocate. Unfortunately, that may not be the case. Children are good to us when we have made a point of telling them the importance of family loyalty and mutual caring. I'll watch out and care for you, but you must do the same for me. It is no wonder that children are often so unconcerned about elderly parents. Most children think that it is the government's responsibility to care for parents, not theirs. It is a shameful belief and it shows that we haven't done a good job of explaining family responsibility.

2) Don't do for children what they can do for themselves. Too many parents do for children many things that they can do for themselves. Teaching children independence is a healthy thing to do. Doing too much for children ends in spoiling children and making them feel entitled. Spoiled children are ungiving and self-centered.

3) Children need our attention some of the time, but not all of the time. We shape our kids. Don't fall into the trap of believing that children will become emotionally deprived if we have our own time and space in life. Many of us grew up in large families where our parents were often too tired and stressed out to pay much more than limited attention to us. We grew up to be decent, loving, responsible and giving adults. Remember that the next time you have the urge to give your complete time and attention to children who have the ability to do a great deal on their own. Love them but don't smother them.

4) The child who doesn't care about us when we hurt is a child we have not raised well. One of our jobs as parents is to help children learn moral and ethical concepts of right and wrong, sensitivity to others, and social responsibility. If you speak to many of the parents of troubled children, you will know that they don't feel it's their responsibility to shape children as caring, responsible, sensible people. That responsibility belongs, they will tell you, to the schools, or the police, or the church. But it is our responsibility and, when we fail, we fail our children and we fail ourselves.

5) Don't give children more than we had when we were children without helping them understand that we've put considerable time, money, and effort into their lives. We expect them to appreciate and to respect our efforts. When they don't, they will receive none of the extra perks of our enhanced quality of life. This important guideline helps explain the uncontrolled materialism of our children in a time when they expect the least affluent of us to buy them toys, clothes, cars and other expensive and often unnecessary items, whether we can afford them or not.

We shape our children, not the next door neighbor. It is our responsibility to teach children the worth of our labor and the meaning of money. If we don't do that, if we feel driven to earn their respect and affection through bribes, then we can expect children to demand greater and more expensive items as time goes by. We can expect children who grow to adulthood still asking us to take care of them.

6) Children without responsibility are children who will feel no responsibility to us. Even in the most affluent of homes, it is important to give children responsibility for the way the home functions. Those responsibilities may include cleaning, washing, shopping, fixing up the home, and a host of things that you may otherwise have to do yourself or hire someone else to do. It's important that children know that not everything is going to be done for them and that they must help out. If they don't know this, they will not learn to value the labor connected with household activities and they will not value our efforts.

This idea of a free ride through life is a growing belief for many children who have been asked to do so little in their own family that they cannot conceive of the notion of work and responsibility to employers. Their lack of involvement at home is often translated into poor motivation to work at a job and often results in job failure. Teach your children about work. Help them learn about responsibility to the family by giving them their share of work to do around the house.

The best time to teach children the responsibilities of caring for themselves and their home is when they are very young. With my daughter, who was then a little more than a year old and who spent half of her time with me and half of her time with her mother during a separation in our marriage, I bought plastic dishes for us to eat from so that she could help wash and wipe the dishes, something she loved beyond reason. When we went shopping, it was her job, even as a little tyke, to pick vegetables and to get the cereals we both ate. She helped vacuum and water the plants, chores she could not get enough of. These responsibilities helped bond us to one another and taught her to help make the home function well.

7) Children learn from us by what we do rather than by what we say. It is no wonder that I became a helper to others. My mother was the neighborhood social worker, the lady who listened to the problems of others and dispensed wisdom and guidance over coffee and assorted pastries. That she was an immigrant woman with a strong accent speaking to mostly Scandinavian women who could barely understand her made absolutely no difference to them. Our neighbors, both children and adults, spent more time in our home than in theirs, it seemed to me. If there was a poor man or woman traveling through town who needed a hot meal, my mother was there to provide it in exchange for work. There were no

free meals at our house. If you were willing to work though, my mother was always there to help out.

My father was a union man deeply involved in the fight to help working people achieve economic independence. He was one of the first people nationally to urge alcohol treatment for the men and women on the railroads, that place of long stretches of boredom and loneliness where large numbers of workers develop drinking problems. He was one of the founders of the credit union movement and a fighter for medical insurance for working people at a time when it was thought to be a communist idea. He knew many of famous politicians of our time and held his head high as a fighter, this little man from Russia with an eighth grade education and a thick accent who, all of his life, worked the back-breaking work on the railroad as a laborer.

More to the point, he was the one who helped the troubled men and women in the union, every Saturday night, when they drank too much or had family fights. He was there for them when a union member killed someone, in passion, and fled to our home for help and guidance. And he gave generously to these men and women from his meager salary. It seemed noble and correct that he should take from us to help others in more need than we were in, an idea that probably sounds corny in these times of cynicism and concern for self.

As a result of the modeling of my parents, all three of their children entered helping professions. Our early sacrifices made us more caring people and better neighbors and citizens. I model these ideals for my daughter, as does her mother, whose early years were similar to my own. She will be a helper too, in her own way, for she has the self-belief and inner-glow which permits her to give to others in ways that are completely selfless. It is a wonderful feeling as a parent to watch this process of wanting to help others develop. It is what Abraham Maslow described as an indication of a self-actualized or complete person.

8) Be involved with your children. By that I mean, show concern and interest in them. Don't use gifts and excessive freedom to make up for a lack of serious involvement in their lives. And, for heaven sakes, don't treat them as if they are your pals. I know parents who allow their children to do just about anything they want to do without feedback or concern. That isn't being a parent. It's reliving your childhood through your children, something that benefits you, not them.

I share these ideas with the men and the women I meet at the coffee shop. They are good listeners and often agree with what I've told them. But they point out that we are in a time when parents have so little impact on their children because of the chaos in our society. Seemingly now, children call the shots not adults, and whatever they want, the society permits them to do.

I don't disagree with that other than to tell them that one parent who holds firm will become two, and then three, until finally, family values and the morals and beliefs of adults who care deeply about their kids and about the word we live in will become the norm. And then, patient reader, kids will be as good again as we know they can be. After all, we were once kids and look at how terrific we are now.

11

Braveheart in the Workplace: Work as Mortal Combat

The Savage And Unfriendly World Of Work

Lila, one of the regulars at the coffee shop, wants to talk to me about her husband. He's just lost his job of 20 years at one of the large firms in southern California who make, or better put, who no longer make airplanes. "He's depressed," Lila tells me. "He has nothing to do. He just walks around the house getting in the way and stuff he never did before. He hates T.V., but it's all he does all day. They gave him three years severance pay and he's close enough to retirement to take it easy for a change, but he doesn't know how."

It doesn't surprise me to hear this kind of story. Men need work. Work gives them something to do with their time. It gives them a place to measure their self-worth and to earn money to provide for their family. Work gives men a schedule to count on. Since men are creatures of habit, you take the schedule away and it feels to men as if they're drowning. Work allows men to be competitive and to express their competence and ability. If men were meant to be hunters and warriors, then work is the place where they are allowed to do battle.

Lila brings her husband in one morning while I'm sitting reading the paper. He's a man in his early fifties, but he looks older. His skin is yellow and his eyes have that blood shot look you see in men who drink too much. They walk over to my table and Lila introduces me to Bill. They ask if they can join me.

After we talk for a while about the small things which most therapists will tell you help people over that initial fear of revealing too much to a stranger, Bill starts to talk about his lack of work and what it's done to him.

"I worked good and hard for them. I was one of the workers who was loyal to the company and helped fight against a union. I supported them every way I could and look what they did to me. I got 15 good years left in me to work and now nobody wants me cause I'm too old. Lila here says for me to relax and take it easy. We got plenty money saved and we can enjoy life. But I don't want to retire. Old people retire. I can still work. If I stop working now, I don't know will happen to me."

I know Bill is right to worry. Men need to work. Money isn't so much the issue. Work is part of how men define themselves. Without work, they men stop having a meaningful role in life.

I tell Bill that I have a friend in the area who needs good workers. It's not a good paying job, but it's work. He looks over at me and shakes his head. "I want a good paying job like I had. I don't want some minimum wage job. That's for Mexicans and kids."

"You've got to start somewhere," I remind him, but he just sits there, his mouth tight and drawn. He's not going to change his mind, even if it means more days of watching TV and drinking. Pride often drives men. Sometimes it drives them to self-destruction.

I see Bill and Lila at the coffee shop once in a while. Bill looks old to me. His eyes seem to have lost their shine. He walks behind his wife, trailing her like a puppy dog.

Work and Sex: Maybe Not in That Order

In the old days, a man's work was a continuation of whatever his father did. Men served their apprenticeships with fathers. Work not only represented a way of meeting basic needs, but it served to continue whatever the family did. Names were often given to signify the family occupation such as, Silverman, Furman, Goldman, etc.

As times have changed, men have often chosen work, not to compliment or to continue family roles, but to exceed them. Now it is important that a son choose an occupation where he will out earn his father or one which implicitly carries more status. The junkman father becomes the attorney son.

The workplace is also where men do battle. Civilized man no longer clubs an opponent to death or skewers someone who makes them angry. What men do now is to apply these combative impulses to the workplace.

Older men often wear out, but young men thrive in the competitive atmosphere of the workplace. And because winning means everything, young men can be devious, harassing, mean spirited and absolutely craven in their desire to reach the top of the heap and, thereby prove that they have the right stuff.

Older men, men more than 45-50 begin to tire of the war games at work. They are increasingly concerned with the quality of their lives. At this point, women begin to outstrip men in the workplace. As men begin a slow decline in their careers, women begin to pass them by.

Many men protest that women are given an unfair advantage in the workplace because of affirmative action, and it's true to some extent. But the reality is that most men cannot sustain their ability to compete in the workplace. At some point they begin to slide. They are also beginning to physically wear out from years of workplace stress.

In its worst form, workplace stress contributes to alcohol and drug abuse, anxiety, depression, marital discord, health problems, and violence against other workers. For years, researchers have known about the connection between spousal and child abuse and problems on the job. A government agency, The National Institute of Occupational Safety and Health (NIOSH) published 3 studies showing the amount of stress in the lives of Male workers. In the first study, one-fourth of the men surveyed viewed their jobs as the number one stressor in their lives. In a second study, three-fourths of men believed that workers have more on-the-job stress than a generation ago. In a third study, problems at work are more strongly associated with health complaints than are any other life stressor-more so than even financial problems or family problems.

This slide from valued worker to someone who is considered obsolete begins to affect men in their middle years. They feel demeaned that organizations so under valued their contribution. The lack of respect for prior contributions as they begin to burn out at work eats away at some men. They often feel dead-ended as they passively view their careers slide downward. The literature calls this a period of low morale and burnout. Much of the reason this happen is because of the way men choose work.

Men often don't choose work because it's what they want to do or what they may be good at but on what will make them the most money or provide the most status. The decline in the way men feel about their work often coincides with the beginning of a mid-life crisis for men.

The Harvard Study is a long term study of the men chosen by their classmates at Harvard to be the most likely to succeed, 20 years after graduation. At age 42, when the study once again looked at these men, it was true that they were the most successful people in their class in terms of achievement at work. It was also true that many of the men viewed themselves as failures. Most had serious marital problems and had been married several times or more. Many of the men in the study had no relationship with their children. Most hated their work and said that they would gladly do something else for far less money. And almost all of them said that they chose occupations to please or surpass fathers, not to achieve satisfaction or personal happiness.

Women, on the other hand, have been socialized to choose work to compliment their interests and skills. When they do well, it isn't for the purpose of proving themselves but because they genuinely enjoy the work.

Helping Men Choose Work Wisely

I've been a university professor for over 35 years now. If there is anything I've learned from the men and women who choose careers it is that career choices made at 18 are not likely to be permanent and that work interests and career goals change. The work chosen early in life by men is not necessarily what a man will do for the rest of his life. You can help the men in your life make better choices in the early years and follow them up with even better choices in mid-career by applying the following suggestions:

1) Help men in your life make career decisions that aren't meant solely to please others. Men may become disappointed in those choices since they may not be what a man truly wants to do. Help men in your life understand their motives for choosing a specific line of work. The best motive is because the man is truly interested in the work. If the money is also good, so much the better.

2) Because a man does something in the early years of his work career, something well paying but very dull, that doesn't mean that he can't change later. Education is one of America's great bargains. Mid-life career changes are not only possible, but they can actually be fun. The happiest people I know are the men and women in my field, social work, who once were in business or who worked at high paying sales jobs. When they tired of the work, they did what they had always wanted to do: to work with people and to help them with their life problems.

You'd be surprised at how many men secretly want to do work we often think is reserved for women such as teaching young children, social work, or recreational work with kids about to get into trouble. At 25, with a new family to support, that type of work may make no sense, financially. But at 50, with nothing to look forward to in a current career, it may make considerable sense.

3) People change in time. What excites someone today may be boring in the future. Don't let a man get depressed over this but help him know that what he now wants is something new and different in his life and that's a positive change.

4) Don't let your man stay with work that bores him. Boredom soon becomes depression. Encourage him to take a chance and try something else. Of course, risks abound, but who said that life was risk free?

5) Finally, there are things other than money to measure success and happiness. Work, which is continually interesting and fun can add years to a man's life and it can also make him a much better partner.

Men and Sexual Harassment

Sexual harassment almost always has the same victim and the same perpetrator. Men are the perpetrators and women are the victims. It doesn't matter what the reality of the workplace might be or how badly women are treating men, or one another, men are usually considered the perpetrators.

Yet we know that people are sexually harassed all of the time. If men in your life are being harassed at work, and over one third of the sexual harassment complaints are now actually men being harassed by female bosses, encourage them to file a grievance and stick to it. Women seem to believe that men want to be harassed. They don't.

One of my students recently told me that he had filed a sexual harassment grievance against a former female boss. She would put her hand inside his shirt and feel his chest or ask him for backrubs on the job. She made frequent statements to him that were overtly sexual in nature and she left sexually provocative notes on his desk.

This would be considered harassment had it been done by a male. For my student, however, the charge was considered frivolous and he lost his job. He's fighting it but that doesn't help paying the costs of family life and school.

If a man in your life is actually sexually harassing someone at work, he obviously has a problem that needs to be treated by a professional. It is a problem as much as drug addiction or violence are problems. And it has to be hurtful to you. Support your man, be fair to him when he is accused of harassment and try to get all of the information possible, but take a stand with him: Sexual harassment is not acceptable behavior to the person on the receiving end or to you. Let him know that in no uncertain terms.

But in this atmosphere of men always being the perpetrator, the following story might help you better understand what goes on in many organizations and the risk men face. Some colleagues of mine met every Friday for drinks in the mid-afternoon. While it wasn't mandatory, everyone from a department met including several female instructors. One of the men with a drinking problem made overtly sexual and very offensive statements, which embarrassed the female instructors. Because the women felt that it was necessary for them to attend the get togethers because they were new and had generally little security, the women endured the insulting behavior for months. Finally, one of them told the chairman of the department that the offending instructor had to stop saying the things he was saying. While my colleague agreed to do that, he didn't do it for reasons we can only guess at.

The female instructors filed a very messy sexual harassment grievance, not just at the offending instructor but also against all of the men who were present at the get togethers. Not one of them had tried to stop the harassment and none had even recognized that it was offensive. All of the men and their families were in danger of losing excellent teaching jobs with great benefits and security because harassment is an offense that can lead to termination. While the wives were all supportive, they made clear that the offending instructor with the drinking problem had to be dealt with. And further, they worked behind the scenes with the administration of the school to help their spouses keep their jobs. Were marriages damaged? I don't know for sure but one of them said to me later:

"Jim can be a real fool when it comes to loyalty. He knew that Tom was going off the deep end, but he never did anything to stop it. He let it happen and I blame him for the disruption and grief in our lives. I support him and I still love him, but he let those women sit and listen to every imaginable sexual innuendo and for that, I'll not forgive him. He was an accomplice and even though he didn't say anything, a part of me believes that he thought it was O.K., and it wasn't. If anything like that happens to your man, it changes the way you see him," she said. "I don't think any of the wives feel quite as secure in the knowledge that their husbands let some drunk insult women for months without so much as lifting a finger to stop it."

And the Ladies Have the Last Word

We've been talking about how tough the workplace can be for men, but the reality is that it's tough for women, too. In a book I wrote about men for helping professionals, I'm reminded of how men and women do better when they band together to make the workplace a kinder environment, by something Stillman (1994) wrote.

> I feel that in the unfettered pursuit of gender politics, women have made a grave mistake in not examining broader issues, such as that of office harassment in general. What men have had to put up with over the years to rise

through the corporate and bureaucratic marketplace, frankly, is as odious to me as sexual harassment. But men have never lobbied against such wage-slave requirements as mandatory lying to cover up company crimes, mandatory company retreats, mandatory obsequiousness toward higher-ups, mandatory cocktails with the bosses brother-in-law, and so on. Maybe they should. However, in their fight against sexual harassment, women have failed to take into account that power always resists challenge, and change is always met with resistance. If women could stop taking the general unfairness of the workplace so personally, they would find allies rather than enemies among their fellow worker-bees." (p.32)

To which the ladies all say, "amen!"

12

Sick, Crazy, and Dying: I'll Never See a Doctor! The Not So Happy State of Men's Health

As you probably know, men do a pretty bad job when it comes to taking care of themselves. They don't exercise enough and their diets are often far too heavy in dangerous fats and alcohol. They see doctors half as often as you do, but when they do see one, they are far sicker and more likely to take more time to heal than women. When they have stress problems, they go for therapy and counseling a fraction of the time that you would do, maybe a tenth of the time. The consequences of this inattention to health are noted in a University of Michigan's Institute for Social Research Report summarized by Gupta (2003):

"Men outrank women in all of the 15 leading causes of death, except one: Alzheimer's. Men's death rates are at least twice as high as women's for suicide, homicide and cirrhosis of the liver" (p. 84). The principle researcher on the study of men's health, David Williams, says that men are twice as likely to be heavy drinkers and to "engage in behaviors that put their health at risk, from abusing drugs to driving without a seat belt" (Gupta, 2003, p. 84). Gupta goes on to say that men are more often involved in risky driving and that SUV rollovers and motorcycle accidents largely involve men. Williams blames this behavior on, "deep-seated cultural beliefs—a "macho" world view that rewards men for taking risks and tackling danger head on" (Gupta, 2003, p. 84).

Further examples of risky male behavior leading to injury and death include the fact that men are twice as likely to get hit by lightning, die in a flash flood, and are more likely to drive around barricades resulting in more deaths by train accidents and drowning in high water. As a significant difference in the way men and women approach their health, Gupta reports that women are twice as likely as men to visit their doctors once a year and are more likely to explore broad-based preventive health plans with their physician than men. Men are less likely to schedule checkups or to follow up when symptoms arise. Men also tend to internalize their emotions and self-medicate their psychological problems while women seek professional help. Virtually all stress-related diseases—from hypertension to heart disease—are more common in men.

American men between the ages of 45 and 64 suffer an estimated 218,000 heart attacks a year, compared with 74,000 a year for women in the same age group, one of many reasons women live more than 7 years longer than men (Drug Store News, 1998). Epperly and Moore (2000) report that men are at much greater risk of alcohol abuse than women with the highest rates of alcoholism occurring in men between 25 and 39 years of age. However, age is not a deterrent for risk factors in men and 14% of men over 65 are alcohol dependent as compared to 1.5% of women in the same age group. Male suicides in men over 65 are 6 times the rate of the general population, according to Reuben, Yoshikawa and Besdine (1996).

These findings of greater health problems among men are not explained by biological differences related to gender. Harrison, Chin, and, Ficarrotto (1988)) write that, "Research suggests that it is not so much biological gender that is potentially hazardous to men's health but rather specific behaviors that are traditionally associated with male sex roles which can be (but in the case of women are not) taken on by either gender."

Saunders (2000) reports that a poll by Louis Harris and associates indicated that 28% of the men as compared to 8% of the women had not visited a physician in the prior year. While 19% of the women didn't have a regular physician, 33% of men didn't have one either. More than half of the men surveyed had not been tested for cholesterol or had physical examinations in the prior year. Waiting as long as possible to receive needed medical care was a strategy used by a fourth of the men studied and only 18% of the men surveyed sought medical care immediately when a medical problem arose.

Additional health data paint an equally troubling picture of male health. Drug Store News (1998) reported the following information for American pharmacists: 1) Women still outlive men by an average of 6-7 years, despite advances in medical technology. 2) The death rate from Prostate Cancer has increased by 23% since 1973. 3) Oral Cancer, related to smoking, occurs more than twice as often in men. 4) Three times as many men suffer heart attacks than women before age 65. Nearly three in four coronary artery bypasses in 1995 were performed on men. 5) Bladder cancer occurs five times more often in men than women. 6) Nearly 95 percent of all D.W.I. cases involve men. 7) In 1970, the suicide rate for white men was 9.4 per 100,000 as compared to 2.9 for white women. By 1986, the rate for white males had risen to 18.2 as compared to 4.1 for women, and by 1991, the rate for white male suicide was 19.3 per 100,000 compared to a slight increase to 4.3 for women (National Center for Health Statistics). In 1991, suicide rates for Black and Latino men were 11.5 per 100,000 or almost six times the rate of suicide for Black and Latino women whose rate was 2 per 100,000. Suicide is the third leading cause of death among African American men. By 2001, suicide rates for all men had increased while suicide rates for men over 60 were from 10 to 12 times higher than suicide rates for older women with men over 85 having an astonishing suicide rate or 54 per 100,000 as compared to women in the same age group of 5 per 100,000 (CDC, 2004)

One of the primary health concerns for men is Prostate Cancer. The National Center for Chronic Disease Prevention and Health Promotion (CDC, 2003) reports that prostate cancer is the second leading form of cancer among men after lung cancer. The CDC (2003) reports an American Cancer Society estimate for 2003 of 220,900 new cases of prostate cancer and that 28,900 men will die from the disease. Most diagnosed prostate cancers (about 70%) are found in men 65 years or older. Because of earlier diagnosis and better treatment, the survival rate for prostate cancer has increased from 67% to 97% over the past 20 years. The prostate cancer death rate is higher for African-American men than for any other racial or ethnic group while the Asian/Pacific Islander group has relatively low rates of prostate cancer incidence and mortality. Among all racial and ethnic groups, prostate cancer death rates were lower in 1999 than they were in 1990. Decreases in prostate cancer death rates during 1990–1999 were almost twice as great for whites and Asian/Pacific Islanders as they were for African Americans, American Indian/Alaska Natives, and Hispanics, suggesting a difference in the use of doctors for early diagnosis, the quality of medical care received, dietary or genetic influences, or taking no action once the cancer was diagnosed.

Harrison and colleagues (1988) believe that as much as three fourths of the seven year difference in life expectancy between men and women has to do with the way men are taught to cope with stress and write,

> Parents assume that male children are tougher than female children, when in fact, they may be more vulnerable than female children. Male children are more likely to develop a variety of behavioral difficulties such as hyperactivity, stuttering, dyslexia, and learning disorders. Macoby and Jacklin (1974) found little in their review of the data to support a view that the early diseases of male children are genetically determined.... Male socialization into aggressive behavioral patterns seems clearly related to the higher death rate from external causes. Male anxiety about the achievement of masculine sta-

tus seems to result in a variety of behaviors that can be understood as compensatory. (p.306)

The Reasons For Male Health Problems

There are many reasons for the health problems of men:

1) Men are far less likely to seek help for physical and emotional problems than women. When they do seek help it is usually at a more advanced stage in the progression of the illness. While men are almost never seen in therapy and counseling unless forced by courts, employers, or spouses, their actual rate of seeking therapy is a third that of women even though they represent fully three times the number of patients institutionalized for mental illness.

2) Men are more likely to internalize stress and convert it into physical problems, substance abuse, or emotional difficulty. To complicate this problem, men frequently live solitary lives with no one to talk to and they find it difficult to communicate feelings with others. When asked why he never came in for therapy after repeated recommendations and referrals by his primary physician, a colleague of mine told me, "I'd rather die than admit to some shrink that I have a drinking problem. In my home you were taught to keep your personal weaknesses and flaws to yourself. I know all about therapy and respect it as a way of helping, but when it comes to me, I can't imagine going to somebody and describing myself as a lush."

3) Men are far more prone to accidents and homicide than women. Part of the reason is due to the dangerous work environments men find themselves in but men take dangerous chances that often lead to serious accidents. As a client once told me, "I know it's pretty dangerous and all, but when I get crazy I drink, and then I drive as fast as I can. It clears my head. Sometimes I go out in my motorcycle and it feels even better. I know it's dangerous, but it works for me."

4) Men often believe that being careful about health is a sign of weakness and that seeing a doctor, unless you are very sick, is feminizing. Men often believe that real men don't listen to doctors or follow medical advice. One example of this is that men are far less likely to finish prescribed medications than women (Kane and Glicken).

5) Heavy drinking is encouraged among men as a sign of masculinity. This behavior is still consistently reinforced by the media and the popular culture, which romanticizes drinking as a way men work problems through. Among some Latino men, to hold one's liquor and keep up with one's peers is expected of macho males. Discussing very poor Latino men, Pena (1991) reports that, "their

code of machismo impelled the men toward cultural behavior that can only be termed destructive. They drank and celebrated with abandon, often with disastrous results, such as bloody fights and vehicular accidents. Almost invariably, alcohol intensified their feelings of machismo and the crudities associated with it." (p 38).

One of my colleagues has a degenerative hip and is in considerable pain. I walked by his office and we talked for a while. I suggested that we have a drink sometime. "Why not," he said, "It's my hip that hurts, not my elbow." Funny story except that I found out weeks later that he'd just been released from a detox program. He called a few days later to set a time for us to go drinking. When I met with him, in fact, he was drinking. He'd convinced himself that he could drink in moderation even though that evening I had to have a cab take him home. Such distorted views of the capacity to drink are quite usual around men. Calahan (1970) says that alcoholism among men is fully 4 times as high as it is among women, although recent findings suggest that the difference is far less than these data would suggest. The author believes that higher rates of alcohol consumption relate to the solitary and isolated lives men lead and to the pressures to achieve.

6) Male babies are far more likely to suffer SID's or other illnesses, which lead to a far higher rate of death among male babies. This data suggest that male babies are more fragile and are prone to serious health problems, a finding which surely contradicts our macho view of men.

From the preceding discussion, it would appear that poor health accompanies men who tend to rigidly define masculine roles, role definitions which often include proving oneself to others. Behavior consistent with rigidly defined masculine roles include higher rates of substance use, unwillingness to follow healthy life styles, smoking, unwillingness to seek help for problems related to stress, and risky behavior including driving while intoxicated.

Coping With Poor Health

An interesting study at Stanford University in the 1970's considered a group of women who had terminal cervical cancer. The group consisted of women who were on the usual treatments following radical surgery including chemotherapy. The average life expectancy for the group was two years. The group was randomly divided in two. Both groups continued with medical care and follow up procedures but one group had weekly support sessions where women were encouraged to talk about their feelings and experiences coping with their cancer.

The other group did not receive supportive sessions. Otherwise, both groups were identical. The women in the group receiving supportive group counseling to deal with emotional trauma related to their cancer lived two years longer on the average than the women who did not receive therapy.

In another interesting piece of research at Menningers Clinic in Kansas, people with essential hypertension (high blood pressure with no known physical cause) were taught bio-feedback techniques (knowing when your blood pressure was high and calming yourself down). In sixteen training sessions, 80% of people receiving the training were able to lower their blood pressures below the levels that medication had achieved, and then they were able to go off medication entirely and maintain lowered levels of blood pressure through the continued use of biofeedback. Bio-feedback was also able to significantly reduce the use of pain killers in people who had severe headaches and back problems, people who often were unable to work because the pain was so severe.

Clearly, there is an emotional component to good health and to controlling the way illness affects your life. When my daughter became diabetic, she went through a period of feeling fragile. Every little ache or pain made her too ill to go to school or her mother or I had to repeatedly go to school in the middle of the day to pick her up. Finally, I told her my approach to illness. Mind you, I grew up with two parents who were legendary hypochondriacs. Watching them, I vowed to never let a preoccupation with illness rule my life. And, by the way, this is the rule of thumb I used with parents whose children were missing too much school when I was an inner city school social worker in Seattle and Chicago. If you have a fever of 101 or more and if you vomit when you stand up then you can stay home for school. Otherwise, you get on with it. If you get sick during the day, you can talk to your school nurse or teacher, but the same rules apply.

Once my daughter knew the rules I enforced, she stopped missing school. Furthermore, she doesn't opt out of activities because she feels badly. Like me, she gets up and does what needs to be done no matter <u>how</u> she feels. She plays tennis with headaches and walks a mile to school when she has the flu. She knows that when you force yourself to get on with it, you usually forget how badly you feel. Being sick, even if you are, is a waste of time. It limits your opportunity for life experiences. So rule of thumb, get on with it even when you're not feeling well, but be wise about it. There are men who are in such denial about there health that they exercise in the middle of a heart attack. That's abject craziness not good mental health.

We know that serious health problems require that you return to the normal routines of your life as quickly as possible. Last year I spent a month in physical therapy getting my shoulder back in shape after surgery for a torn rotator cuff, the result of years of competitive tennis. I went back to work within days of the surgery because work is necessary for me to function well. Getting back to work, even when you are not quite ready, speeds up the healing process.

When I was perhaps five, my mother developed bronchial asthma, an illness that plagued her until her death. It's likely that she had a post-partum depression after the birth of my younger brother and that the depression turned into asthma. In those days we knew little of the impact of depression on illness. Rather than treating the depression with therapy and a mild mood elevator, my mother was placed on an experimental drug known as ACTH. I can still remember how excited we all were when she responded so rapidly and got better. What we didn't know was that the drug was an experimental form of cortisone, a powerful new steroid and anti-inflammatory. I discovered that her doses of ACTH and the resulting doses of Cortisone were 200 times the dose we would use now.

Steroids can poison the body when used too much. In time, my mother's health deteriorated so badly that she spent much of my childhood and adolescence in the hospital. The steroids damaged her cardio-vascular system, caused arthritis, distorted her facial features, damaged her spinal column causing her back to arch. Worst of all, the drug cause her to become highly paranoid. For years before her death, she imagined that people were listening to conversations through holes they had made in the floor or wall. On a plane thirty thousand feet in the air, she would whisper because someone she knew from home might overhear her.

I watched my mother become increasingly ill and, increasingly depressed and withdrawn. I am convinced that no one spoke to her of getting well but, instead, did to her what Seligman describes as teaching the patient to be helpless or, creating "learned helplessness." Rage against illness, fight it, make it your enemy. Know it well, know it as well as you know yourself, and then fight it with everything you have so that it doesn't get the best of you.

From a considerable amount of experience working in medical social work in hospitals, I believe that recovery from an illness requires, a) getting back to normal activity as quickly as possible; b) confirming what doctors tell you through your own research; c) understanding that there is a great deal of validity in folk cures like chicken soup and hot tea with honey if you believe that they will be helpful; d) recognizing that we all have our own ways of handling illness and, if it works, use it. I was back to hitting a tennis ball a month after surgery. The doctor told me that I was crazy but the exercise improved my outlook on life and I took it easy. Two days after surgery, I drove myself to the beach even though my arm was in a sling. It probably wasn't very safe, I'll admit, but being disabled is a state of mind and it's not in my mind to define myself, or anyone else, as disabled.

Part of my professional career has been spent working with serious disabilities at Sister Kenny Foundation in Minneapolis and the Rehabilitation Unit of University of Washington Hospital in Seattle. You see the people who come in with a serious disability (paralysis from the neck or waste down) and die in few months because they've given up. Physically, they ought to be healthy, but spiritually and emotionally they are dieing from the moment they became disabled. And then you see the fighters, the ones who get in there and work their tail off and tell you that they'll walk, by god, and nothing you can say or do dissuades them. In time, they may walk a little, but it is the fighters who get on with their lives. The quitters just curl up into fetal positions one night and you find them dead in the morning. Never give up.

Drugs and Alcohol

Drugs and alcohol are problems that are everything they're cracked up to be in the lives of men. The data on alcoholism suggest that problems with liquor may be as high as 15-20% of the male population and that drugs add another 5%. Some researchers suggest that many men who are not alcoholic go through overdependence on alcohol in times of stress and that the problem is far greater than the data suggest.

Unfortunately, men are socialized into the world of substances. Being a man means that you can drink a great deal, that you <u>should</u> drink a great deal. There is great romance about drinking to most boys who think that, along with smoking, drinking puts you in the fast lane to manhood. Men often romanticize alcohol and think that it's perfectly alright to use it whenever they are stressed out, happy, mad, or in need of a lift to bolster their courage. Most crimes are committed while men are intoxicated. Alcohol is a killer. Almost 100% of the reason alcoholics and heavy drinkers die relates to the use of alcohol.

How do you know when a man has a drinking problem? Several simple indicators can be used. 1) He has a drinking problem if the thought of not having a drink fills him with anxiety. 2) He has a drinking problem when he knows that it will be difficult to stop drinking, even for a day. 3) He has a drinking problem if he is missing work because of hangovers or if he's drinking on the job. 4) He has a drinking problem if he overstocks liquor for fear of running out. 5) He has a drinking problem if the urge to drink liquor is greater than the urge to eat. 6) He has a drinking problem if he began drinking in his pre-teen or teenage years and the amount and frequency are steadily increasing. 7) He has a drinking problem if it takes progressively more liquor to give him the desired effect he wants. 8) He has a drinking problem if his short-term memory is affected by drinking. 9) He has a drinking problem if he is developing secondary sexual problems like impotence as a result of your drinking. 10) He has a drinking problem if his life revolves around drinking.

There are a many things that you can do to help men who have a drinking problem. The research that had hoped to show that a heavy drinker might, with training, become a social drinker, has not panned out at all. Drinking is an addiction that seems not to be treatable like other addictions such as obesity, where you can help people continue eating but at reduced rates. Drinking is an addiction that physically challenges the drinker to stop once he's begun to drink. For most drinkers, it is very difficult to stop because the physical and emotional addictions are so powerful.

Some writers believe that men prone to alcoholism have genetic reasons that make stopping very difficult. Other writers believe that the livers of alcoholics are different and that alcoholics are able to drink more than normal drinkers before they become ill. Finally, many writers conclude that families of origin provide some men with positive messages about alcohol that reinforce alcoholic behavior. We also know that certain cultures are likely to give both positive and negative messages about alcohol, which serve to limit or enhance drinking. Most studies note very low alcoholism rates among Jewish and Asian people, for example. And finally, some alcoholics become addicted to alcohol as a way of coping with stress.

There isn't much romance in the treatment of drinking. Nothing very easy to make the process simple. You must stop drinking first. This is usually accomplished by a either a short stay in a residential facility taking two to four weeks, outpatient treatment, or joining a self-help group like alcoholics anonymous and learning the 12 step philosophy. There are new medications that seem to be helpful in achieving abstinence and limit depression which sometimes accompanies the end of heavy drinking. If you have been a very heavy drinker for a very long time, you may experience the D.T.'s. This is a temporary neurological disorder caused by eliminating alcohol from your body. You may have chills, nausea, hallucinations, painful headaches, aches in the body, spasms, and convulsions. This is why it's so important to be in a facility equipped for physical reactions when anyone quits drinking, although most people who quit, do it on their own. As you can tell, doing it on your own can have dangerous repercussions. But listen to a typical story from a former client about his drinking history.

"I've been drinking for as long as I can remember. I think I probably started by stealing booze from my parents. It was never a big deal in my family. There was always a lot of booze around. Nobody seemed to miss it. You could say we were a drinking family. Booze was an important part of the day for my mother and dad. You could see this look of sheer joy come over their faces when they started to drink after work. It was intoxicating to me. I could hardly wait to start. When I did start, it was every bit as good as I'd imagined it would be. I can close my eyes and think of the first drink I ever had, it was that good. I guess I was drinking pretty heavily by my twenties, although I was proud of the fact that I had it in check. It never interrupted my work or my day. It was like a side thing. I was always a happy drunk too, so no one knew how much booze I was into each day, but it was easily a fifth or more.

"I got married and had kids, although the whole thing is a blur in my mind. By my thirties, it was beginning to affect me. I was drinking on the job and I was having more bad days than good ones. Lots of violent hangovers. Maybe by then I was adding a couple of bottles of cheap wine to a fifth a day. It didn't matter anymore what I drank. I'm not proud of it but I've put away stuff you're not supposed to drink like shaving lotion and anti-freeze because it had alcohol in it. Then one day my boss confronted me about my drinking and it all fell apart for me. My family couldn't stand me, I had no friends, I was in awful shape physically. I went on a binge, and the next thing I knew I was in a county facility with all the street drunks. Bums. Of course, I was one of them, too, but my pride wouldn't let me believe it until I was well enough to get to know them. I was a year or two away, at best.

"I took the treatment seriously, although, like most drunks I've had my relapses. You can't drink again. No way. Once you start, you can't stop. But anyway, I've been pretty successful at staying off booze. My family won't have anything to do with me anymore, of course. I still have no friends except for the people from A.A., and an alcoholic is always a potential enemy, never a friend. I'm thirty-eight and my doctor says the drinking has ruined my body and cut my life span. He says that most alcoholics can't work past fifty, there's so much damage to the body. I hope he's wrong. I'm trying to stay in shape and eat right. It's tough. For a whole lot of years, I never ate a full meal. The booze was my food." And another story from a friend:

"I had what I thought was expensive taste in liquor. I figured that anyone who drank expensive liquor didn't have a drinking problem. I was very ritualistic and formal about my drinking. I never drank before five and never drank so it affected my work. No hangovers or getting sick at work. I was a hot shot money man. Big decisions, big rewards. Had to be clear headed. Lots of guys were using drugs because the signs were so unclear then. You had a runny nose, no one suspected cocaine. Must be allergies. It's in the air, everyone would say if they saw someone sniffling. I was actually drinking a bottle of very expensive Scotch a night. At thirty bucks a bottle it was no financial burden, not like the cocaine users who were sniffing hundreds of dollars a day away. I felt pretty sanctimonious, I can tell you.

"One day I woke up and there was blood all over the pillow from a nose bleed. I didn't think much of it, but it started to happen a lot and so I went to my doctor. He took my blood pressure, which was off the wall and immediately guessed about my drinking. Drinking drives up the blood pressure, I discovered. He said I was in immediate danger of having a stroke. That I had overloaded my body's ability to cope with the alcohol and if I didn't stop, I'd die. They hospitalized me right away. I didn't die, but as I was coming off the booze, I had a series of minor strokes. My memory isn't sharp anymore so I can't do the big money making stuff. I have a slight slur in my speech so sales aren't the thing anymore. I sell shoes. Yessir. That's what I do. Straight salary, no commission. I could make more in one day on commission in my old job then I make in a year doing this.

"I don't know why I started drinking like I did. My folks were never big drinkers. I think I liked the romance of drinking expensive liquor. It was like sitting at home in this fine place I had and enjoying the hell out of my life. Like the Lord of the Manor. How better to do it than to toast the world with a drink. Now I get to toast the world with a glass of fruit juice. I may have more strokes. No one can say for sure. You live for the day, I guess. If you don't, it can get pretty depressing."

While drugs are less of a problem than alcohol in America, they still present a significant problem for men. And by now, we should all know that there is nothing truthful about the term recreational drugs. All drugs, however benign they may sound, hold potential risks for users. The synthetic drugs like crack cocaine are the most dangerous because we know little about their quality or potential potency. Drugs, like alcohol, are extremely addicting and are very difficult to stop using. Consider this story from one of the regulars at the coffee shop:

"I was working construction the summer everybody seemed to be using drugs on the job. Some guy would come down in the morning with his little stash and by noon, we'd all be high. I'd hate to have lived in the building we did that summer. Everyone was so wrecked I can't imagine that it was worth a damn when it was done. We'd use everything. A lot of us had been in Nam so we were pretty sophisticated about drugs.

"Anyway, one thing led to another and before I knew it I was at the V.A. for detox. I started having tachycardia attacks. You know, when the heart beats really fast. Also, I was becoming really paranoid. I started picking fights with guys on the job for reasons I can't quite figure out. I thought it was smarter to do drugs than booze. Booze wrecked my daddy bad. It's not smarter. Drugs will kill you just like booze, only quicker. I still crave them. The same type of guys come around on the job to sell you drugs but we got the union to keep them away. I'm not sure I could stop myself from buying. Lots of the guys feel the same. Drugs will kill you. I don't care what kind they are or how little you take them, they'll kill you. In Nam, more men got messed up on drugs than because of fighting. It turned a lot of guys into zombies."

What Can We Do To Make Men Healthier?

Getting men to initiate contact with their physicians, following through on medical advice, and maintaining healthy lives is a task everyone should strive to help men achieve. My suggestions for good male health are: 1) Don't separate physical health from emotional health. 2) Help men keep good information handy regarding their health histories and the histories of their parents and siblings. 3) Find doctors who treat men with respect and are sympathetic to the needs of men. Men have better rapport with these doctors and will listen to them and accept their advice. 4) Help men stay in shape by working out or walking with them. 5) Be certain that meals men eat at home are healthy and low in fat and carbohydrates. Discourage fad diets or diets that haven't been discussed with a physician. 6) Help men become free of addictions to alcohol and smoking. 7) Don't let men ignore signs of health problems. This may mean going with them to see doctors. 8) Be sympathetic but firm when men deny health problems. 9) Help men stay on medical regimens, but be careful not to nag. 10) Be aware of health changes and point them out even if a man is in denial and doesn't want to discuss it. Again, be sympathetic but firm.

Men are in serious difficulty these days. We should all work to keep men healthy so they can continue to be the partners to women and the parents to children who lose men to illnesses that are not only curable, if caught early enough, but are also preventable.

13

Dangerous Men: Men Who Abuse, Batter, and Destroy Women

Every one of the women who meet regularly at the coffee shop and most of the men have had experiences with abuse. By fathers or brothers, by mothers or sisters, by husbands wives and ex-lovers. Not one of them can say a good thing about the experience. To be physically or sexually abused is one of those life traumas in that some of us never recover from.

One of the men I see at the coffee shop from time to time walks by my table a few times one early morning during the summer smog. It's a time when Southern California looks as if its been sprayed by a soot machine. When he gets enough courage, he stops by my table and asks if he can join me. He introduces himself as Paul. Paul beats around the bush for a while and then asks about what to do if someone, unnamed, has a problem with their temper.

"What sort of problem?" I ask.

"A problem that when they drink too much, they hit their wives and children," he responds.

"Tell me about it."

"I don't know if I can," Paul says. "When I drink, I can't control my temper. I get very angry at little things and I take it out on everybody around me."

"Why are you wondering about it now?" I ask.

"Because my wife reported me to the police and they're threatening to put me in jail if I don't get some help."

I nod. I'm too tired to let him know what I think of men who abuse women and children or his lame excuse that it's the drinking that sets him off. Like most abusive men, his abuse has been going on for a long time and his wife and children have probably suffered his bad behavior in silence. It's a silence that's seldom broken because the families of abusive men often collude in their misbehavior for reasons I will explain.

"I think the police are right, Paul. I think you need some good help to control your temper. Men who beat up on women and children have problems, Paul, and the best way to deal with those problems is to get some good counseling."

Paul looks over at me and I notice that his eye is twitching. "Hell," he says, "my lawyer said to get someone to testify in court for me. I was gonna ask you to do it."

"I'm sorry, Paul, but I don't do that sort of thing. When men hurt others, they need help," I tell him, "not somebody to get them off."

Paul is angry now. He thought that I would lend a sympathetic ear because I write about men, but he's wrong. I am utterly unsympathetic to abusive behavior and he gets up, mumbling, and leaves. One of the regulars tells me later that he felt like punching me in the face. All of the men I talk to later sympathize with his plight. "An ungrateful wife," someone says. "He puts food on the table and she calls the police on him." Like too many men, they fail to understand the incredible damage abuse can do: to body and to the spirit, damage that may last forever.

While much of what we call domestic violence is thought to be done by men to women and children, women do their share of abuse. Half of the violence to children in America is done by women. Men seldom report spousal abuse but a variety of studies peg the number at levels almost as high as male abuse of women. But because I am writing to help women who know first hand about violence to the body and to the spirit, I can share a few findings on the men who abuse.

We know a lot about abusive men. We know that they tend to have been abused as children. They are often pathologically jealous and have low opinions of women. Abusive men have a tendency to deny the pain they cause. When confronted by the broken jaws or the damaged eyes they inflict on others, they deny that it ever happened or somehow believe that wives or children are to blame.

We know that many abusive men have a limited ability to express feelings and often use violence to convey the dark emotions building up inside. And we know that abuse is most likely to occur when men drink or use drugs.

Abusive men believe that women are very likely to be unfaithful, a belief that is used continually to justify the pain they inflict on their wives and girl friends. We know that abusive men and abused women frequently come together in relationships so violent that it is difficult to explain the damage they do. In some bizarre way, abuse becomes a way of expressing love for many of these couples.

What should we do? So little real research has been done on the treatment of abusive men that no one really knows. We have good evidence from studies done in Minneapolis and Duluth that immediately taking the abusive man to jail and charging him with abuse tends to dramatically lower additional episodes of abuse. We also know that among a minority of men, perhaps 15% to 25%, jail tends to escalate violence and that these men are the ones who stalk, threaten, and sometimes kill women.

Because we only have the word of the couple that the abuse has stopped, it's difficult to know what, if anything, works in counseling. But from the research I have been doing on abusive men, a pattern seems to be evolving.

While men usually hate the idea of therapy and counseling and only infrequently use it, when counseling is done with men in groups of other abusive men, the group seems to be able to modify the abuse. Perhaps this is because the men in the group serve to become what Robert Bly calls, "Men of Wisdom", the good substitutes for absent or abusive fathers.

We know that change takes a long time, perhaps six months to a year or more. Approaches that help men handle anger and develop feelings of repulsion for their behavior also seem effective. We know that we can help men use language instead of violence to express feelings of anger. And we can teach men to take "time outs," to walk away from violent feelings when they might use force.

When violence exists, separating men and women physically is often necessary. Retraining orders need to have teeth in them and the police need to be advocates for abused women and children who must often face the abusive man alone.

Finally, we know that abuse is serious and that intervention, no matter how much the couple may not want it, can save lives. Being proactive rather than waiting for the abuse to cycle into something unmanageable can prevent terrible harm to the body and the spirit.

To get to how we can stop abuse, maybe it would help to understand the reasons men abuse their women and children.

<u>The Reasons for Abuse</u>

1) Many abusive males have, themselves, been physically abused by parents, caretakers or other family members. The physical abuse frequently includes sexual abuse. Data would suggest that roughly 65% of the men who abuse women and children have, themselves, been abused.

While it might seem odd that an abused child would grow up to abuse others because the experience would, hopefully, have sensitized him to the dreadful ramifications of abuse, the dynamics are such that unconscious rage often directs the behavior. One client of mine told me that he was so angry that every encounter with another human being left him throttling an impulse to, "Hurt somebody real bad. I never knew why I was so mad all the time but I was and somebody was going to pay for it that was for sure."

2) This need for payback is often reinforced by other men in the abuser's life who believe that physical abuse is the best way to keep women and children "in line." This distorted view of reality is continued on by the choice of what Robert Bly (1986) calls, "Men of Wisdom." Men of Wisdom are the father substitutes whom abusive men choose as their primary source for advice, information and guidance. Because these Men of Wisdom, themselves, have abusive patterns, the abuser not only finds his abuse reinforced, but he may be criticized for not being abusive enough. In truth, the abuser may believe that his abusive behavior is far too mild because his man of wisdom ridicules his behavior as being meek.

3) Abusive men are frequently insensitive to the pain they inflict. When one asks them about an abusive episode, they understate the harm done. They deny hearing bones break or believe that the victim is the responsible one since they should not have been sitting the way they were when they were struck. Or the abuser will tell you that the victim should have seen that the abuser was angry and removed themselves from the situation.

Many abusive men believe that victims like to be abused and, therefore, the abusive man is only fulfilling the wishes of the victim. When x-rays are produced which indicate that harm has been done, all too many abusive men will argue that the victim had a congenital weakness in the area damaged or that they were not struck that hard.

4) Abusive men are often pathologically suspicious and jealous. This view of women may be a reaction to the passive roles mothers took when the abusive male was, himself, abused, or it may represent the view of the men who abused them when they were children. Male abusers see infidelity everywhere. A new perfume or a nice dress may prove to the abusive male that a spouse or a girlfriend is sexually involved with someone else. Minor breaks from routine are sure signs of infidelity to these pathologically suspicious men.

Some writers believe that abusive men are so incapable of intimacy that distrust of the motives of women are translated into fear of love, affection, and intimacy. To allow someone to love you is to invite terrible psychic pain. To avoid the inevitability of such pain, abuse is a way of negating women through reducing their emotional impact on the abusive man. Ridicule and emotional abuse go hand in hand with the physical abuse. Abused women are often encouraged to be as physically unattractive as possible. When women fail to comply with the need to minimize attractiveness, the abuser may make certain that his abuse helps to accomplish this through physical beatings.

Some writers also believe that multiple pregnancies serve the abuser's wish to keep women from being attractive to other men, although this doesn't stop abusive behavior and many women have been abused during pregnancy. Abusive men may encourage weight gain in women as a further way of keeping women unattractive. Multiple pregnancies may serve to define the abusive man's masculinity. This attempt to negate attractiveness of a wife or girlfriend is further assured by the abusers infidelity. Many abusers will report that they have affairs as preemptive strikes to guarantee their emotional safety when wives or girlfriends "inevitably" become unfaithful. The abusers belief in the inevitability of infidelity is true even when women become so emotionally and physically scared that they no longer have the emotional strength to seek other men. And the more the woman becomes unattractive, the more the abusive man ridicules her looks to further discourage her from seeking other men.

This view of women as deceivers also characterizes the abuser's view of children. Abusive men believe that children are yet another group who potentially will hurt them if they care too much. Much as the abuser endured <u>his</u> abuse silently, children are expected to endure theirs in the same way. Abusers further the destructive impact on children by encouraging them to believe that the abuse is good for them and that it will build moral character. It is not unusual for abusers to join groups that believe in the innate evil of all people. These groups justify the use of pain in exorcising evil from children. So disassociated are abusive men from children, that they generally sever contact with them in divorces, angry that they have supported children financially and that children have chosen, or been ordered, to live with mothers or other care givers. In their view, children, like women, are unappreciative and take from men without giving anything back.

5) A great deal of abusive behavior comes in the midst of substance abuse. Substances not only give abusive men the courage to abuse, but they permit the release of repressed rage. For the victim of abuse the abuser may appear irrational in his outbursts. However, often the abuser is more in touch with the abuse he suffered as a child under the influence of alcohol or drugs. This may not be a conscious memory as much as a reminder of feelings of powerlessness and rage. Abusive men who use substances are at their most dangerous when they are intoxicated or high. Not only are they less able to control their rage, but they are

operating in states of altered consciousness in which prior abuse to them creates feelings of powerlessness that strengthen rage reactions.

The wife of an abusive client told me: "He could be the most charming man who ever lived when he was sober, but get a drink in him and look out. He'd kick the dog, then he'd beat on me and then, if the kids were around, he'd whack them pretty good. Something happened to him when he drank. It was like he changed personalities. He was a monster, really. Just an awful, abusive crazed monster when he drank."

6) Abusive men often have extreme difficulty using language to convey emotions, desires and expectations. When victims do not do as abuser's desire, hitting or ridicule are the ways abusers have been taught to deal with anger since they also distrust language. For them, words are signs of weakness. When they do use language that conveys feeling, the experience makes them feel oddly effeminate and unmanly. Language that causes emotional harm to others is perfectly OK and many abuse victims say that the worst thing about the abuse is the terrible things said to them by the abuser. In general, men, they believe, use action and not words to convey desires. Not surprisingly, these men use violence in other arenas of their life including work. However, to a surprising degree, abusive men may be seen as mild-mannered and calm elsewhere, reverting to abuse and tyranny only in the safety of their homes.

7) Because abusive men hate the feeling of powerlessness that comes when they try and talk out issues which trouble them, talking therapies are notoriously ineffective in reducing violent behavior. Therapy often makes abusers feel as powerless as they felt when they were abused. As one of my clients told me, "This thing we're doing (talking about abuse) makes me more angry and depressed than I ever was. I remember all the terrible things that happened to me. I hate coming here. I know I have to, but I hate it."

8) Abusive men need to control the women and children around them. This need to have others comply with their wishes is a way of preventing unfaithfulness and deceit. When women and children fail to comply with the abusive man's demands, the result is generally abuse. Abusers often see failure to comply with increasingly confusing and minute expectations as sure signs of deceit. Frequently, they test women and children by making expectations so unclear that failure will surely result. Failing tests of loyalty reinforces their negative view of women and children.

9) Abusive men train those whom they abuse. Abused children often abuse others or move into abusive relationships where they are the victims of abuse. These patterns, while dysfunctional, are normal to victims. Often the cycle of

abuse is reinforced by male abusers who encourage grown children to use abuse with their own children. Generations of violence may be perpetuated by a single angry man with poor skills at containing rage.

10) Many writers report that abusive men feel remorse after an episode of abuse. The term, "Honeymoon Period" is used to define the remorseful period in which, out of guilt, the abuser becomes warm, loving, and tender. Abuse victims describe this period as the time when their lives are the happiest. Like other reinforcers, the victim is addicted to these moments and may put up with continued abuse because it often results in a short period during which relationship is at its best. Some men suggest that these periods are short-lived because victims encourage additional abuse so that they can move back into honeymoon periods. While this may occasionally be true, it is more likely that the rage inside abusive men has a limited period in which it can lie dormant before outbursts of anger take place again.

The Impact of Abuse on Victims

There is strong evidence to show that abusive male behavior has a particularly bad effect on women and children. Those negative effects, both physical and emotional, are as follows:

1) The high probability that children who watch domestic abuse or, are themselves victims of abuse, will abuse their children and spouses. As an abused friend of mine said to me once about what his abuse as a child did to him, "You're hypervigilant. You think everyone and everything out there is intent on doing you harm. You fight the impulse to strike back all of the time. It's a struggle just to get through the day without hitting back. My ex-wife said that the chip on my shoulder got bigger and bigger as the day went by. She was right. By the time I went to bed, I could hardly even think about sex I was so suspicious, up-tight, and angry."

2) Victims of male physical abuse are far more likely to enter into relationships with people who have been abused or who will abuse them. This fact almost always assures the continuation of male violence in relationships. The probability of this is so great that workers in the abuse field have come to expect it.

A former client explained this tendency when she told me, "You love those whose behavior is predictable. You grow up in a healthy home without violence, you're intimate with men who don't use violence. You grow up in an abusive home, you look for people who will abuse you. It's your crazy read on what love is, to be abused."

3) Victims of male physical abuse are often also sexually abused.

4) Physical abuse of women often moves into physical abuse of children. This may be explained by the man's increasing rage, which cannot be well managed in the home and transfers itself on to anyone and anything in the home the male can hurt. Abusive men may also experience sadistic joy in abusing animals or in taking treasured personal items from women or children. Abuse may also include destruction of property, delight in ridiculing, and special pleasure in making others feel as helpless and as powerless as the man felt as a child when he was abused.

5) The spouses and girlfriends of male abusers are very likely to suffer severe physical problems including repeated broken bones, scars, disfigurement, burns, cracked and out of aligned jaws, problem pregnancies because abuse may continue on during pregnancy (about one fourth of all pregnant women report being battered during their pregnancy), loss of hair, broken noses, loss of sight, and a host of disfiguring and dangerous physical problems which result from the battering.

6) Spouses and girlfriends of abusers are often emotionally scarred by the abuse. They suffer from depression, withdrawal, loss of self-esteem, substance abuse, loss of employment, mental illness, and a host of serious emotional problems related to continued physical battering and the verbal and emotional abuse that accompanies abuse.

7) There is considerable evidence that child abuse is one of the leading causes of death and disfigurement of children in America. The amount of child abuse is roughly even when gender is considered. However, because men are stronger physically, the damage done to children by men may be greater than that done by women and, consequently, children battered by men may have more serious physical problems. Those problems may include loss of sight, brain damage, severe disfigurement particularly when hot fluids have been used or battering is repeated in the same physical area, loss of the use of limbs, paralysis, and deafness (ears and eyes are special targets of abusers).

8) The emotional harm to children who have witnessed domestic violence or have themselves been victims include life long depression, rages which translate into panic and anxiety disorders, substance abuse, underemployment or difficulty working, sexual disorders, low self-esteem, prostitution (85% of the prostitutes who have been interviewed have been physically and/or sexually abused), and continued rage reactions and difficulty controlling anger. Children who have been physically abused are very likely to physically harm other children, as well.

Children from highly abusive families exhibit depression and find it difficult to think through problems. They may suffer from low self-esteem and self-awareness and have problems identifying feelings. Many abused children show extreme hypersensitivity that turns into adult paranoid suspiciousness and manipulativeness, traits that often characterize the adult male abuser.

Getting Help

If you are in an abusive relationship, you need to seek professional help as quickly as possible. Sometimes that help includes withdrawing from the abusive man by going to a shelter for battered and abused women. Other times that help may include reporting the abuse to the police and having a man enter mandatory treatment or face a jail sentence. Don't let a man abuse you. It will lead to emotional damage, physical and health problems, and in too many cases, permanent disfigurement and death.

14

Changing Male Behavior

Men seldom use counseling and therapy as a way of changing troubled behavior. There is something about the process of therapy that is far too feminizing for most men. Therapy asks men to be introspective, a process most men find difficult and troubling. Therapy asks men to share highly personal feelings, something men have been trained not to do. Therapy asks men to trust another person when men are often unable to even trust those who nurtured them and the spouses and girlfriends who now love them. Therapy asks men to be sensitive to others, but men often believe that as providers and care-takers, that women and children are insensitive and unappreciative, and that sensitivity to others has no reward.

However, authors by the name of Robertson and Fitzgerald believe that therapy can be helpful if it's supportive, reinforcing, instructional (advice giving), and non-confrontational, and write,

> counseling psychologists need to offer programs that emphasize self-help and problem-solving rather than offering solely counseling for deeper insight into self-development and personal emotions. Our findings are consistent with the tradition in counseling psychology that encourages the use of culturally sensitive formats for providing services to clients representing ethnic minorities and those designated as "special populations." Although it is not usual to think of men in this fashion, it is also true that the masculine mystique generates a unique assumptive world that appears to function as a barrier to men in many areas (e.g., emotional, psychological). (Robertson and Fitzgerald, 1992, p. 245)

In a study of the willingness of men to talk about feelings and to discuss their emotional life, Robertson and his colleagues (2001) report that while men may be unable to answer questions posed to them about their emotional life, they readily answer questions that involve problem-solving, task-completion, and structured activities. The authors suggest as alternatives to spoken responses to questions about feelings that men do better when given written assessments and structured educational assignments. However, men with lower levels of gender stress are perfectly able to effectively discuss emotions. The authors found that stress is one of the most common problems men want to discuss in treatment and that 80% of the men in their study readily participated in a discussion of the best ways to relieve stress. The authors suggest that focusing on physical and emotional awareness of stress may lead to changes in behavior and attitude. One of the common problems with many forms of therapy is a failure to recognize that when men enter therapy, they are experiencing forms of physical discomfort (anger, anxiety, depression, stress, and confusion). As the therapy is focused on the relief of these physical discomforts, the client feels relief and there are probably bio-chemical changes as a result. The man who <u>feels</u> better will continue on in treatment because there appears to be a direct link between therapy and the relief of symptoms. When men go to doctors, if they don't feel better after seeing a doctor they either see someone else or they see no one and try and handle the problems on their own. Telling a man that he might feel better months down the pike is the same as inviting him to leave the office.

There are other ways of helping men. The rest of this chapter discusses some practical ways we can help many of the men who experience serious problems in their lives.

<u>People Of Wisdom</u>

Robert Bly believes that men seek other out other men for advice and support. He calls these men, "men of wisdom". They listen well, are empathic and sensitive and possess expertise in solving certain types of problems. We gravitate to these people because they help us through informal means that can be very helpful and reinforcing. Sometimes they do the very things that good therapists do and they are blessed with kindness and good judgment.

My father was a man of wisdom. For 50 years he was involved in the union movement in North Dakota. It wasn't only that he was ideologically tied to the union and believed that united workers were stronger in their fight against management, he also believed in reaching out to co-workers and helping them in time of need. Our Saturday nights were often spent with men and sometimes their wives coming to our home to discuss a range of problems with my dad. Some of the men came just to borrow money to drink but usually they came to talk. My father who was a non-believer in therapy and who used to mock psychiatry became an excellent therapist. Because of my father a number of men and their wives ended up in drug or alcohol treatment. He saved the careers of man men who got into trouble on the railroad because they damaged equipment, themselves, or others while intoxicated.

When I was a young man working the graveyard shift on a switching crew in North Dakota, it was my dad who accompanied the police when they came to pick up a crew member who earlier in the evening had killed a man he thought was having an affair with his wife. My dad's presence didn't surprise anyone. Later, when the man was released from jail, it was my father who got him back on the job. Whenever I rode the trains to school or to California to visit my sister, or any of the adventures I had as a youth thanks to a railroad pass which allowed free access to the second tier trains of America, there was always someone in any town or city waiting on the platform, calling me Sammy(My dad's name) ready to buy breakfast or to help in a thousand ways because my dad had helped that person in the past. Over 50 years you accumulate a lot of friends. My dad was a man of wisdom, a natural helper in a time of non-professionals who reached out to the men and women of America, a poor immigrant Jew in a non-Jewish place doing work Jews seldom did who was embraced for what he clearly was: A man of substance and wisdom like so many other wise men who have come before and after him, a man to help others.

Helpers like my father should be given roles in our society. In the workplace, they might be identified as people with good common sense who listen well and who offer good advice. These men and women of wisdom should be given a special role in the workplace to offer men the very thing they need desperately but fail to seek: a helping experience to move them in more positive directions in their lives.

Where therapy can be far too formal and structured for many men, the person of wisdom may offer a service so gentle and informal that it appears to be little more than offering a sympathetic ear. This form of service is well within the boundary of what appeals to many man who hurt. It saves them the embarrassment of a formal contact with a therapist while still providing the needed help.

In the lives of men, few men model positive, affirming behavior. As we learned in the material on abusive men, often the advice given violent men by other violent men, reinforces abusive behavior. The person of wisdom, however, could be the man to counter these negative influences.

Men Helping Other Men

Men don't join movements or groups for the most part. The process of being part of a group feels foreign to them. A sports group or a group to deal with a task might be O.K., but a therapeutic group would be an unlikely alternative for many men. And yet, the literature suggests that when men change, that it's often because of a group experience.

This recognition of the power of groups has encouraged a number of therapists to use groups when dealing with men, particularly when men are in legal difficulty and are required to seek treatment. Many diversion projects for spousal abuse and domestic violence use mandatory groups to treat men in jeopardy of doing time in jail. The results are mixed, of course, primarily because of poor record keeping by clinicians and the limited research to date. While we can't say with assurance that groups are the answer to male problems because a large number of men drop out when the going gets tough, emotionally. yet groups seem to help many men. Perhaps what we need is some use of groups in a less obviously therapeutic way. For example, work groups in which quality control and productivity are key ingredients, perhaps such groups have a therapeutic impact on men. Perhaps men who go to sporting events or bars with a regular group of friends use the group interaction to work through problems which they would otherwise not deal with. Perhaps the groups that men gravitate to are chosen at some level for their supportive and therapeutic nature.

Men develop friendships out of shared experiences. Friends become the tennis and golf partners, the co-workers, the bar hoppers. Men, unlike women, do not set out to be friends. They set out to do tasks together. In the course of those tasks they talk to one another. A good deal of the time the talk is about private issues. There is no resolution of the issue because men respect the need for other men to resolve problems in their own private way. It is a process that looks indirect and seems disconnected, but to men, it makes sense.

Between breaks in a tennis match, men will talk about their work or their children. They make statements about the emotional pain they're in and they'll go for a beer, ostensibly to cool off, but in reality, to finish unfinished personal business. It's the way men operate. They don't think of their friend's problem as something to challenge their friendship. They think of talk as a natural outcome of being together and if the talk is personal, so what?

As I write this, my tennis partner, a world famous academic, has been asking to play on the weekends, something he's never been able to do in the past. He's said nothing about marital problems but I guessed that something was wrong just by his availability. I've never violated his privacy by asking him directly about his problems. It would be an unseemly thing for a man to do, particularly since our relationship is specifically limited to playing tennis.

Yesterday, our match was canceled by rain and we saw a movie and then had dinner together, the first time we've done something like this in five years of playing tennis together, 4 and sometimes 5 times a week. In the course of having dinner he began to discuss a job offer from another university. I wondered what his wife thought and he matter of factly said that he wasn't sure that she would come because they were not living together anymore.

I wasn't surprised about this information and had, in fact guessed it months earlier. I wasn't surprised that the matter evolved as it did, either. Nothing so personal as a failed marriage would ever be an initial topic of conversation. It would be discussed when the right time came and in the form of a trial balloon. If the other person responded, fine, but if he doesn't, no harm done.

My tennis partner kept saying that there were tennis courts all over the place and that it was only a short flight to his new school, as if this was about tennis and not something much more important. Tennis had become his ballast now. Not me, you see, but the ritual and the schedule of tennis was keeping his life intact. He could not tell me about his pain or the dilemma of a failing marriage so near the end of his career. No, all he could manage was to figure out how his rituals would remain if his marriage failed. And telling me a little about his marital problems made sense since this was about tennis and not about personal pain.

I respect this attempt to maintain privacy in the midst of pain. It is the stoic aspect of men that is so intriguing and heroic. A friend can help, you see, but in the indirect ways which help a man maintain his life. Don't tell me what to think or do, says the man in difficulty, just help me do the things I'm used to doing so I can that I can keep myself together.

Some people, me included, think that many more men should be made to accepted into counseling and therapy programs. Social work, for example, the largest professional group to offer counseling and therapy services in the country is almost exclusively a female profession. Not so much because men don't apply but because they often unwelcome and uncomfortable in female dominated professions. That's really a shame because boys need male role models. When men are in school settings as teachers and social workers, developing male problems can be dealt with and resolved before they get out of hand. Boys listen to and respect male advice and direction.

<u>On Changing Our Lives</u>

Many people think that there is something magical about therapy and the many theories that explain how people change their lives. When all is said and done what therapy does is to look logically at problems and then, in an equally logical way, developing strategies to deal with each issue confronting you.

That may sound simplistic, but that's what finally happens. To be sure, the road to change may have its bumps and potholes, and getting up the energy and wisdom to make correct decisions can take time, but in the end, men control their lives just as you do. You decide how you want to live your life, what you like and don't like, the problems that trouble you most, and the emotional problems that follow you year after year. No therapist can do magic. They can nudge, and explain, and confront, and sympathize with you and your feelings, but in the end, you make the decision to change.

There are clearly issues from the past that cause our path to health to be filled with detours. Certainly our parents leave us with legacies of unresolved issues and beliefs and can cause confusion and pain. Sometimes it's difficult to get over a particularly troublesome crisis or life event such as a painful marriage or a tragedy. Health problems can legitimately keep us from our journey toward self-discovery and emotional health.

All of these current and prior life issues are part of life. We are aware that they affect us but we needn't become slaves to what has happened in the past. What is done is done. Our job is to get on with our lives and to never succumb to the temptation to blame others for our current problems or to think that if something hadn't happened, we'd be so much better off.

In reality, our lives are shaped by many events and certainly, we can't say that problems early in our lives are the reason for the problems we now experience as adults. Many people have early life problems, some of them traumatic and gut wrenching and they become healthy and productive adults. With that in mind, let's consider some guidelines to help us direct our lives in positive ways.

Rule One Of Getting On With Your Life: Never blame other people for your problems. Never assume that because something was done to you when you were younger, that it must forever continue to bother you as an adult. Blaming others for our problems is great fun, but it doesn't make the problem go away. As a matter of fact, in study after study the one approach to therapy that seems to be the least effective in changing people's behavior is the Freudian approach, which tries to show connections between past events and present behavior. There is compelling evidence that this approach may, in fact, cause people to become even more emotionally upset. The effective therapies are straight ahead therapies that help us see a problem as rationally as possible and then logically develop strategies to resolve the problem. As one of my former clients told me at the end of his therapy experience:

"You used to tell me that it wasn't what people did to me that made me angry and upset, it was the way I thought about those people. I could understand what you were saying in my head but I could never quite make it work for me. Then last week my boss said something rude as he always does and instead of getting angry at him I thought, what a rude bugger and what problems he must have to treat people the way he does. I didn't get mad, I felt sort of matter of fact. I can't tell you what a sense of power it gave me to not blame him and, in the end, not to get angry. I control how I feel about things. It's great to have such control."

Rule Two: Calling yourself a victim or defining yourself as someone in recovery is a great excuse for not dealing with your problems. You might be a victim and you might be in recovery, but defining yourself in these ways serves to keep your attention off change and on what was done to you. Unfortunately, all too many writers are focusing on this aspect of healing because it makes for catchy titles and it sells books. But, in a sense, we are all in recovery over something: ill-health, a bad marriage, hurtful relationships, abusive parents, bad job choice, unemployment, etc. If you view yourself as someone in recovery, you never get on with your life. Instead, you focus endlessly on the thing you are getting over.

You don't define yourself by what is wrong with you but rather, you define yourself by what is right, what works, and the things you are most proud of. Listen to a friend define himself to see what I mean.

"If anyone came from a dysfunctional family, it was me. There was more craziness in that family than anyone could ever believe. My mom and dad were at each others throats every minute of everyday. All of us kids had major problems from bed wetting to stealing. You couldn't talk about anything at home without someone making fun of you or calling you names. It was crazy as hell. But you know something, along with the craziness there was a lot of sanity. We were taught to be tough and self-reliant. We stood up for one another when we had to. We all learned to see our poverty as something which didn't make us bad, just poor. And in the end, we all did well in our lives. Really well. Sure we have problems, who doesn't? But I listen to people talking about dysfunctional families and I shake my head. Dysfunctional is in the eye of the beholder. All I know is that if anyone had called our family dysfunctional, my old man would have kicked him out of the house. We were a lively family, he'd say. We had opinions. We liked to argue. So what? Exactly, so what?"

Rule Three: Therapy is for short-term issues, it is not forever. Neither is therapy a substitute for doing the day to day work you must do to change your life. Many people substitute therapy for a social life. They use therapists or support groups as substitutes for the friends and loved ones they should be developing on their own. Therapy is to be used for the emotional blocks that we cannot remove by yourself. Therapy is hard, upsetting work. Its purpose is to get you to see connections between your life decisions and your current behavior. When you enter into a therapeutic relationship, be prepared to work hard. Using therapists to socialize with or to complain to is not what therapy is about.

Therapy is also expensive. It may, depending on where you live, cost up to $150 an hour. There are a number of problems, such as generalized anxiety and mild depression that may be very nicely handled by a brief course of medication. Sophistication of medication for mood changes is very high, at present. Many of the new drugs appear to be quite safe and may offer relatively quick relief that therapy is not able to offer. Therapy is not a panacea. You should know that before you go into it, and be sure to check with your physician who may have other ideas about why you're feeling as you do. Remember, many diseases cause behavior to change. Always see your physician before going for therapy to make certain that you haven't a particular type of illness that may cause behavioral changes.

A friend of mine had been suffering from generalized anxiety for several months. He wondered if he needed therapy for some underlying emotional problem. A simple blood sugar examination discovered that he was suffering from adult onset diabetes. With proper glucose control, the anxiety went away. Another friend sought therapy for a mild but particularly resistant depression that just seemed to linger above the surface no matter what insight she had in therapy. A wise therapist began to suspect a physical reason for the depression. Sure enough, a thyroid test indicated that her thyroid was depressed. Proper medication eliminated the problem quickly.

Rule Four: No one said that life would always be sweet. Sometimes life is just plain terrible. You ride out the storms without criticizing yourself for the times that aren't so great. I know that isn't always easy and that we all have a tendency to get down on ourselves when things go badly, but everything you've heard about depression and anxiety is true. The more we get down on ourselves for not having perfect lives, the more prone we are to self-hate, anger, and worry. My personal equation for happiness is that out of seven days, two are terrific, one is bad, and four are fine enough so that I feel neither terrific nor awful. Of course, more good days are always a plus.

Rule Five: Many people in our lives tend to give out negative messages. Don't listen to them and, certainly, don't believe them. If they give out messages that are especially negative, try to understand their reasons but limit the contact with them. No one needs downers in their lives, particularly you.

There are people who have never learned to give positive messages. They catastrophize and worry about everything. A friend tells me that his wife is that way. He doubts, he tells me, that she's had a happy or joyful day in her life. Whenever she feels happy, she throttles the feeling by telling herself that something awful is about to happen and she had better prepare herself for it. To be happy will just weaken her ability to cope with the awful thing about to happen. "She is one of the great downers of my life," he reports. "She has many fine qualities and is a loving and a tender wife, but whenever it comes to having fun, she doesn't know how. If I'm in a playful mood, she cautions me that I'm not preparing myself for the realities of life. She always has a story or two about the person who felt just as I did and then something awful happened to them. Any catastrophe like the Oklahoma bombing of the federal building or 9-11 is a sure sign that you can never be prepared enough for a tragedy.

Her mom is the same way so I know where she got it from but, my god, it can be maddening. She won't travel because she knows an accident will happen. She has what I call "Block House Mentality" like the survivalist who live with their guns and their dogs awaiting the end of the world. When it ends, what good will being prepared do for anyone?"

Rule Six: Have your own goals in life. Be certain of them and then stick to them no matter what other people say to try and dissuade you. Most of the time, that is. If your goals are off center, getting you into trouble, impractical, or pie in the sky, have the foresight and strength to change them.

Jim Schefter, my old high school buddy tells me that in his work as a professional writer: "If you let people constantly berate your work, it's impossible to be successful. I find people whose opinions I value. I know that the feedback they give me will help my work because it is always positive while still being direct and useful. I don't think any of us can keep up a body of work when other people are constantly berating us. To do the work I do as a writer, I need to have a vision of myself and absolute confidence in my ability. You may call it a dream, Morley, but for me it's a capacity to work. I've had moments in my life when other people are banging away at my confidence. In time, it gets to you. So I look for positive people to be around. The good they say and do is a great motivator to do better and better work."

Rule Seven: It's not what happened to us in life that may cause us to be unhappy, it's how we view these life occurrences. The Greek Stoic Philosophers believed that people had the ability to control their emotions by what they said to themselves about an event. That's why people who go through really unfortunate life problems often come out of the event better than they were before the event. As a professor who teaches and writes about crisis, the research is very interesting on the subject of the way people cope with personal crisis. The Chinese symbol for crisis also means opportunity. Many people who go through horrible life events come out of these events happier, more fulfilled, and better integrated human beings. To a person, they indicate that this is so because they reevaluated their life as a result of the crisis and were able to chart new and healthier directions. Once again, it isn't life events that makes us unhappy, miserable, and feeling awful, it's the what we tell ourselves about the events.

Therapists such as Albert Ellis and Rudolf Dreikurs have been able to show us that people talk to themselves about the issues they face everyday. Based on what they tell themselves about life events, they are calm, concerned, angry, depressed, or miserable, you name the emotion. Here's an example of the way we talk to ourselves and how it may affect us emotionally:

Let's assume that we're on the eighteenth floor of a building attending a meeting. There is only one door leading in and out of the room. Windows and an eighteen story fall are the only other ways out. A small dog walks into the room. We may be curious, annoyed, or amused by the dog because each of us perceives the situation differently. That is, our self-sentences may tell us about the situation in ways unique to us.

Now, instead of a small, cute dog, lets say that a huge, very mean looking Doberman Pincher walks in, foaming at it's mouth, a frenzied look in it's eyes, and growling in a distinctly scary way. To a person, I suspect, that we would all tell ourselves that we are in the midst of extreme danger. There is no way out and the possibility is high that we might get mauled. The emotion, which results from our perception of the situation is very likely to be fear or extreme apprehension. We perceive a situation, make judgments about that situation, and then tell ourselves in simple declarative sentences the information that allows us to make objective decisions. It's that simple.

Following that bit of logic, if we have the potential to say things to our self that cause us to be anxious and afraid, we also have potential to say things to our self that are comforting and positive. The trick is to view the situation rationally and calmly. In that way, we are able to understand the situation and then to seek solutions in a logical and systematic way before we act. This approach is particularly useful for men who often want to get to the core of an issue as quickly as possible, resolve it, and then get on with life.

Rule Eight: In the end, it isn't the college degree you have, or the amount of money you've accumulated, or the successes that you've had in life, it's the experiences you've accumulated, the knowledge you've gained, and the positive and productive way you've approached your life. Everything else, it seems to me, is ground noise that neither makes you happy nor gives you a jolt of good feelings when you think about it. To be sure, there are people who gloat every day over the money they've accumulated or the titles and degrees they've achieved. Most of us, however, get that glow of good feelings when we consider what we've done with our lives. The better we've used our time and the more positive experiences we have had, the more likely we are to give ourselves high marks for leading successful lives.

And the Ladies Have the Last Word

Rachel, one of the women who joins us from time to time, has just had an epiphany about her life. She tells us, "I started going to church a few years ago, just a small church near my house. It can be very comforting, you know, to be around other people when you're feeling down. And I guess that's what I've been feeling since my ex and I split up. Anyway, this pastor, he said something, I think it's from the Bible. He was talking about love and he said that real love would come to all of us, and then he said, 'I sought him whom my soul loves and, you are altogether beautiful, my love, there is no flaw in you.' I thought, what beautiful things to leave church with. I've been feeling good since, and I think you're right, Doc. It's not what happens to us, it's how we see it. We had good years together, me and the ex, and instead of remembering that, I've been thinking about the bad times and beating myself up. I don't think I'm going to do that anymore."

Everyone looks a little wistful. Rachel has captured the meaning of being positive and we all feel a sort of glow as we file out of the coffee shop to face the day.

15

And the Ladies Have the Last Word Again

I'm sitting at the coffee shop one morning reading the paper when several women walk up to my booth and ask if they can talk to me. As far as I can tell they've never sat in on one of our groups before. One of the women introduces herself as Rhonda and the other says her name is Sarah. I motion for them to sit down and join me. They sit for a while looking at nothing in particular and then they settle down and tell me that they have loving men in their lives. "I know you've been helping some of the ladies with problems they have with their men," Rhonda says, "but we want you to know that our men are wonderful. Not all men are bad men." I nod my head in agreement. "And the thing is," Sarah says, "we know a lot of nice men, men who are good to their wives and kids and we just wanted you to know that there are good men out there." We sit for a while in silence and Rhonda says, "I think my boys are going be good men, too. They're good kids and they listen and are respectful, and they make my husband and me happy to know we've done good by them."

How odd, I think, that women have to assure me that their men are good. Many men would bend over backwards to praise their wives, but we live in strange times and this need to affirm that all is well is part of a growing reaction to male bashing and the unkind way men have been portrayed in the media. Maybe it has to do with the war in Iraq and 9-11 when, in times of danger, men keep us safe. I don't know but it seems to me that we've gone through a very long period of male bashing. I hope we're done with it. It demeans everyone.

It also seems to me that men are beginning to appreciate women more than ever. I hope I'm right about that because men have treated women badly for a very long time and it's shameful when I think of the abuse that goes on in the homes of America by ordinary men who think that women are punching bags.

I hope the sex wars I've experienced during my lifetime won't result in the same type of gender conflict I'm beginning to read about in Japan, where young Japanese men and women are increasingly staying at home with their parents, not having relationships or getting married, and having their intimacy needs met superficially by friends. This trend has so lowered the birth rate, that Japan's population will begin to decline by 2006. Sexual activity in Japan is dead last among developed nations and the children who should be having mature romantic relationships are now being called "Parasite Singles" because they mooch of their parents, maintain themselves on menial jobs, and declare to everyone, <u>Kekkon Shimasen</u> (I won't get married!).

After the two ladies leave, the old regulars come by and show me some wedding pictures of a child's wedding. The mother and father look proud and happy and there's a glow about the way they look. Is there anything more loving and tender than two mature people in love? One of the ladies says, "You should have come, doc. There were some nice looking ladies and I'll bet even a couple of them might have found you interesting. Women love bald men, ya know?" Well, I don't know about that, but I'm sure I would have had a good time because even with the conflict I've been writing about, when men and women are good together, they can be very good. What could be better than finding love at a mature time in your life when you have the wisdom to appreciate it?

So, ladies, and maybe the few gents out there who have read this book, I do wish you well in the future. I hope you've learned a little about men and about yourselves, and that you can use what you've learned to make your life a happier one.

God bless!

Morley Glicken

About the Author

Dr. Morley D. Glicken is the former Dean of the Worden School of Social Service in San Antonio; the founding director of the Master of Social Work Department at California State University, San Bernardino; the past Director of the Master of Social Work Program at the University of Alabama; and the former Executive Director of Jewish Family Service of Greater Tucson. He has also held faculty positions in social work at the University of Kansas and Arizona State University. Dr. Glicken received his BA degree in social work with a minor in psychology from the University of North Dakota and holds an MSW degree from the University of Washington and the MPA and DSW degrees from the University of Utah. He is a member of Phi Kappa Phi Honorary Fraternity.

Dr. Glicken published two books for Allyn and Bacon/Longman Publishers in 2002: The Role of the Helping Professions in the Treatment of Victims and Perpetrators of Crime (with Dale Sechrest), and A Simple Guide to Social Research; and two additional books for Allyn and Bacon/Longman in 2003: Violent Young Children, and Understanding and Using the Strengths Perspective. He published Improving the Effectiveness of the Helping Professions: An Evidence-Based Approach to Practice in 2004 for Sage Publications and Working with Troubled Men: A Contemporary Practitioner's Guide for Lawrence Erlbaum Publishers in 2005. He is completing Learning from Resilient People, and, An Introduction to Social Work, Social Welfare Organizations, and Social Work, both to be published by Sage Publications in 2006.

Dr. Glicken has published over 50 articles in professional journals and has written extensively on personnel issues for Dow Jones, publisher of the Wall Street Journal. He has held clinical social work licenses in Alabama and Kansas and is a member of the Academy of Certified Social Workers. He is currently Professor Emeritus in Social Work at California State University, San Bernardino, and Director of the Institute for Positive Growth: A Research, Treatment and Training Institute in Los Angeles, California. The Institute's website may be found at: http://www.morleyglicken.com and Dr. Glicken can be reached online at mglicken@msn.com

978-0-595-36007-9
0-595-36007-6

Lightning Source UK Ltd.
Milton Keynes UK
30 November 2010

163618UK00002B/182/A